Beating the Blood Sugar Blues

Thomas A. Lincoln, MD
John A. Eaddy, MD

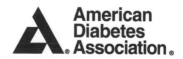
American
Diabetes
Association®

Director, Book Publishing, John Fedor; *Editor*, Sherrye Landrum; *Production Manager*, Peggy M. Rote; *Composition*, Circle Graphics, Inc.; *Cover Design*, Bremmer & Goris Communications; *Printer*, Transcontinental Printing.

Printed in Canada
1 3 5 7 9 10 8 6 4 2

The suggestions and information contained in this publication are generally consistent with the *Clinical Practice Recommendations* and other policies of the American Diabetes Association, but they do not represent the policy or position of the Association or any of its boards or committees. Reasonable steps have been taken to ensure the accuracy of the information presented. However, the American Diabetes Association cannot ensure the safety or efficacy of any product or service described in this publication. Individuals are advised to consult a physician or other appropriate health care professional before undertaking any diet or exercise program or taking any medication referred to in this publication. Professionals must use and apply their own professional judgment, experience, and training and should not rely solely on the information contained in this publication before prescribing any diet, exercise, or medication. The American Diabetes Association— its officers, directors, employees, volunteers, and members—assumes no responsibility or liability for personal or other injury, loss, or damage that may result from the suggestions or information in this publication.

⊗ The paper in this publication meets the requirements of the ANSI Standard Z39.48-1992 (permanence of paper).

ADA titles may be purchased for business or promotional use or for special sales. For information, please write to Lee Romano Sequeira, Special Sales & Promotions, at the address below.

American Diabetes Association
1701 North Beauregard Street
Alexandria, Virginia 22311

Library of Congress Cataloging-in-Publication Data
Lincoln, Thomas A., 1924–
    Beating the blood sugar blues: proven methods and wisdom for controlling
    hypoglycemia / by Thomas A. Lincoln and John A. Eaddy.
       p. cm.
    Includes index.
    ISBN 1-58040-048-5 (pbk. : alk. paper)
    1. Hypoglycemia. 2. Diabetes—Treatment—Complications. I. Eaddy, John A.
    II. Title.

RC662.2 .L56 2001
616.4'66—dc21
                                      2001022773

Contents

Foreword

One of the most vexing problems for diabetic patients is dealing with hypoglycemia. This is especially true for insulin-treated patients. In the Diabetes Control and Complications Trial (DCCT), excellent blood glucose control resulted in a dramatic reduction in microvascular complications—those involving the small blood vessels, especially in eyes and kidneys. Progression of retinopathy was reduced by 70%, microalbuminuria (protein in the urine as a sign of kidney disease) was reduced by 39%, and clinical albuminuria by 61%. Yet, in the DCCT, people who maintained excellent control of their blood sugars also experienced a three-fold increased risk of severe hypoglycemia (requiring assistance of another person) and of hypoglycemia resulting in seizure or coma. What should a person with diabetes do to minimize the likelihood of hypoglycemia happening? There are no easy answers.

Two people who have a lot of personal experience with diabetes—110 years between them—are Dr. Thomas Lincoln and Dr. John Eaddy. During that time, they have had lots of hypoglycemia. And from their experiences, they have learned how to adapt their lives to be successful in dealing with the inevitability of hypoglycemia, and reduce the impact of it. They have done this, too, without sacrificing good blood glucose control. Now, in this book, they share their wisdom and their experiences with us. Remarkable for their clarity and their insight, Dr. Lincoln and Dr. Eaddy come alive to us in this book. They can teach you how to adapt to hypoglycemia so you can go on about your life. There's a lot of good advice here.

Jay Skyler, MD
University of Miami

About the Authors

Thomas A. Lincoln, MD, has had insulin dependent diabetes for 63 years, since age 13. He received his MD degree from the University of Minnesota Medical School and is Board Certified in Preventive Medicine (Occupational Medicine). He has been Medical Director of the Health Division of the Oak Ridge National Laboratory, Corporate Medical Director of the Union Carbide Corporation, Member of the American Board of Preventive Medicine, and a consultant in occupational medicine. Because of his lifelong personal experience of living and working with diabetes and people who have diabetes, he has counseled hundreds of people about how to live and work with hypoglycemia. Although retired, he continues his interest in the education of people with diabetes. This book is his latest educational effort. He enjoys classical music and opera.

John A. Eaddy, MD, has had insulin dependent diabetes for 49 years, since age 12. He is Board Certified in Family Medicine. Currently he is professor emeritus in the Department of Family Medicine at the University of Tennessee in Knoxville.

Since 1980 he has taught other people with diabetes, their families, and many health care professionals about intensive self-management of diabetes. His teaching emphasizes how to live well with diabetes and minimize the risk of disabling complications. He is also on the staff of the University of Tennessee Diabetes Center and the Tennessee Camp for Diabetic Children. He enjoys canoeing, hiking, classical music, world travel, and working outside in nature.

Acknowledgments

Many people have contributed in various ways to this book. We are especially grateful to diabetes patients and their families who gave us information about their experiences with hypoglycemia and the special ways they attempted to prevent or manage it. We also gratefully acknowledge the support and encouragement of our wives. Our survival has literally depended on their continuing concern, emotional support, and their rescues during hypoglycemic crises. When we became discouraged and depressed about the slow progress of our book, our families stood by us until we got back on track again.

We thank our original editor, John Cameron. When the prospects for publication were dim, he continued to contribute his time because he felt that this was material that people with diabetes needed to see and understand. He has recently been diagnosed with type 2 diabetes, so he now has a special personal interest in the topic. He has been patient with our stubbornness and has helped us make our presentation more readable for the general public.

We appreciate the support of the American Diabetes Association in selecting this book for publication, and thank Sherrye Landrum, our editor, for her help.

Introduction

Hypoglycemia (low blood glucose) is a common problem for people with diabetes who take insulin or certain oral diabetes medications, such as sulfonylureas. When you strive to keep your blood glucose levels near normal, you are more likely to experience low ones, too. In fact, hypoglycemia is one of your most important treatment problems. This book was written to help you with this problem. We have both had long-term insulin dependent diabetes, with 110 years of combined experience between us. Our purpose in writing this book is to explain the many factors that influence your blood glucose level and how to deal with them. We offer you suggestions on how you might prevent too frequent episodes of hypoglycemia—the first of which is: always work closely with your health care provider on controlling your diabetes.

Your goal, as you live with diabetes, should be to keep healthy and avoid serious complications later in life due to your disease, and that means trying to keep your blood glucose nearer to normal levels. Modern life is often too hectic for you to follow a rigid schedule of diet and exercise and expect the same insulin dosage to work every day. Our book gives you general guidance, explanations, and personal philosophy so you can live an almost normal life while keeping your blood glucose near normal levels.

Chapter 1 gives an overview of hypoglycemia. Chapter 2 compares the relatively low risks from having occasional hypoglycemia with the much more serious risks from allowing your blood sugar to remain chronically high. Chapters 3 and 4 emphasize the importance of checking your blood glucose and keeping a careful record of those numbers and other factors that might affect your blood glucose. These are the clues that can help you figure out how to avoid low blood sugar levels in the future. If you develop hypoglycemia so severe that you need assistance from relatives or friends, chapter 5 gives details on how they can help you treat it at home. Chapters 6, 7, and 8 describe the roles of insulin, diet, and exercise in avoiding severe hypoglycemia. Chapters 9, 10, and 11 discuss the concerns of children in school, teenagers, and adults. Chapter 11 is concerned especially with the effects of hypoglycemia on sexual activity and pregnancy. Chapter 12 gives advice on how to avoid the most worrisome problem for most diabetics— having severe hypoglycemia while asleep.

You need to be concerned with the possible severe consequences of driving while hypoglycemic. Traveling also poses special risks. These situations are covered in chapters 13 and 14. Chapter 15 cautions on the special dangers of alcohol consumption for those of us who have diabetes, while chapter 16 discusses the possible effects of other medications on your diabetes control. Some less common but nevertheless very important effects of hypoglycemia on your nerves and vision are described in chapter 17. The psychological effects of hypoglycemia are covered in chapter 18. People who have had the disease for many years often become less sensitive to the symptoms of hypoglycemia and, therefore, are less aware that their blood sugar is declining. Chapter 19 discusses this rather common problem. The book ends with perhaps the most important chapter because it is about you assuming responsibility for managing YOUR OWN diabetes.

The book is organized to help you find the information you want. Your diabetes educator and people at your diabetes clinic can explain passages in this book if you want to know more. If you have a computer and know how to access the Internet, there is a huge amount of information available on diabetes. A good place to start is the Web page for the American Diabetes Association (ADA) located at http://www. diabetes.org. See the section titled: "Getting Information about Diabetes on the Internet." If you do not have access to a computer, you may send a letter to American Diabetes Association, Inc., 1701 N. Beauregard Street, Alexandria, VA 22311 or call 1-800-DIABETES (342-2383).

An Overview of Hypoglycemia

I n this book, we discuss the effects on people with diabetes of too little sugar (glucose) in their blood—hypoglycemia. The basic problem in controlling blood glucose is that you only eat food at various times of the day, but your body uses energy continuously—at about the rate of a 100-watt light bulb. When you are walking, it is about twice that. If you are performing hard work or vigorous exercise, it may be 500 watts. Your brain consumes energy more or less at the constant rate of a 20-watt bulb. When you eat a meal, your body must store the energy from the food and then release it as it is needed during the day and night.

In nondiabetic people, blood glucose stays between 60 and 160 mg/dl whether they have just eaten a big meal or haven't eaten for 12 hours. One of the jobs of your pancreas is to keep the level of glucose in your blood in the normal range by releasing one of two hormones (glucagon and insulin), in response to a change in blood glucose levels. When blood glucose falls too low, the pancreas releases glucagon, which signals the liver to release stored glucose, bringing the glucose level back up. If blood glucose rises above normal, the pancreas releases insulin, so it can help body cells take in the blood sugar and burn it for energy, bringing the high blood glucose level back down.

Diabetes results when your pancreas cannot do its job. The pancreas of people with type 1 diabetes no longer makes insulin. They must inject insulin to help their body use glucose, and they must eat to raise blood glucose when it gets too low. The pancreas of people with type 2 diabetes continues to make insulin but not enough or their bodies cannot use it well. People with type 2 diabetes treat the disease with meal planning and exercise. They may also need one or more types of diabetes pills to bring blood glucose back to normal levels. About 40% of people with type 2 diabetes move on to using insulin at some point for better glucose control. Some diabetes pills can cause hypoglycemia (low blood sugar), but people who use insulin are most likely to have it.

When you have taken too much insulin or you have used up glucose faster than normal in work or exercise, your blood glucose may fall low enough to cause you problems. People have a variety of symptoms depending on how rapidly the blood glucose falls and how low it gets. However, you will find these symptoms vary from time to time and will change over time. You need to be aware of your usual symptoms and stay alert for any new signs that hypoglycemia is developing.

> What does 60 mg/dl mean? Most people do not understand what these numbers mean in terms of everyday quantities, such as ounces and cups. A milligram (mg) is about the weight of a postage stamp, and a deciliter (dl) is about a half a cup. To say that the normal range of glucose is 60–160 mg/dl means that there is between 1 and 3 teaspoons of sugar (glucose) in a gallon or so of blood.

Symptoms

When your blood glucose falls below 60–70 mg/dl, your body reacts by releasing adrenaline from the adrenal glands (located above the kidneys). This emergency action raises blood glucose a small amount as a defense against hypoglycemia. Adrenaline also causes unpleasant effects (called adrenaline symptoms), including a rapid pulse, sweating, and nervousness (Table 1-1). These symptoms may fade after you have had diabetes for years.

The brain is very sensitive to low blood glucose. As glucose falls, our thinking functions begin to fail—even doing simple addition, reading the newspaper, or writing a check become difficult. The symptoms produced by falling blood glucose are often called brain starvation symptoms and are also listed in Table 1-1. As your glucose falls lower, some of your muscles will fail to work properly. You may become slow and unable to write or walk steadily.

Causes of Low Blood Glucose

Here is a list of the factors that contribute to your risk of developing hypoglycemia. These factors are discussed in later chapters.

1. Unplanned exercise
2. Missed meals or snacks
3. Problems with glucose monitoring
4. Too much alcohol
5. Delayed or uneven absorption of injected insulin
6. Changing insulin needs during the night
7. Drugs interfering with recognition of hypoglycemia
8. Breakdown of the body's natural glucose-balancing processes

TABLE 1-1

Symptoms of Hypoglycemia

Adrenaline Symptoms

Anxiety	Nausea
Nervousness	Paleness or flushing
Hunger	Sweating
Rapid heartbeat	Chest pain or tightness
Tremor	

Brain Starvation Symptoms

Moderately low blood glucose	*Extremely low blood glucose*
Tiredness	Loss of coordination
Slowed mental function	Slurred speech
Confusion	Feeling cold
Muscle weakness	Paralysis of extremities or face
Blurred or double vision	
Mood changes (giddiness or anger)	Involuntary muscle contractions
Dizziness	Seizures
Headache	Unconsciousness
Bizarre behavior	Coma
Numbness or tingling (lips, tongue, nose, extremities)	

The Risks

In children (but rarely in adults), if hypoglycemia lasts for hours or gets severe enough to cause a coma, permanent brain damage or death may occur. Clearly, it is vital to prevent hypoglycemia in children. Fortunately, most adults recover from severe hypoglycemia with no major long-range effects. But you might be tempted to avoid hypoglycemia by letting your blood glucose levels run higher than normal. Please consider that the long-term consequences of high blood sugar can be devastating. Allowing your blood sugar to run high dramatically increases your risk of complications, such as blindness, kidney failure, nerve damage, and circulatory problems that lead to heart attack, stroke, and amputations. So, you may find yourself thinking that you are between a rock and a hard place. But hypoglycemia is, by far, the smaller problem, and you can control it with good diabetes management.

Good Management Practices

If you want to control your diabetes and also prevent hypo-glycemia, you must check your blood glucose before each meal, at bedtime, and at any other time you need to know if you are high or low. You need to keep honest records of your blood glucose checks and use them to try and understand why your blood glucose was at the level it was. This understanding can help you avoid going too low in the future. It is easy to shrug your shoulders and say, "I think I am doing what my doctor says to do. My high (or low) glucose level is his fault. He's not giving me proper directions." That's unfair. You, and you alone, are in charge of your blood glucose levels. Try to understand the meaning of each blood glucose reading. Did you eat too much? Did the meal have more carbohydrate in it than you realized? Is this a new food that you've never eaten before? Did you take too much insulin? Did you take too little insulin? Did you take it too early? Did the walking you did earlier have an effect on your blood sugar now? Has your sore throat and cold also affected your blood sugar level?

Understanding the rise and fall in blood glucose levels is difficult for everyone—patients, families, educators, and health care providers. No one has all the answers. The only way to learn is to spend a few moments after each blood glucose check and try to analyze why it is where it is. At first, depend on your providers to help you learn, but don't get lazy.

There's something new to learn every day. If you have low blood sugar every day at about the same time, you can learn to avoid it by making changes in your diet, exercise, or medications. It's a balancing act, and you are the ringmaster.

Treatment of Hypoglycemia

The treatment of hypoglycemia should be simple. All you need to do is to eat food that can be quickly digested and converted to blood glucose. Once your brain gets enough glucose, it will stop complaining and rapidly return to working normally. However, if you are sleeping or you are under the influence of alcohol or drugs or just watching TV and not paying attention, you can miss the earliest symptoms of hypoglycemia.

If every time your blood glucose fell below 50 mg/dl you had a throbbing headache, being aware of hypoglycemia would be simple. However, headache is rarely an early symptom. There are so many variations of even the usual symptoms that it is useless to try to list them all. Many people with diabetes say that each experience is a little different. Because the early symptoms are subtle, busy people ignore them until they get into real trouble. How to treat your own hypoglycemia is covered in chapter 5, but we discuss some basic principles here.

Start treatment early. When you are concerned that your blood glucose is dropping low and you can't check your blood glucose level, eat something. Even if you can check, it may be wiser to eat first and then check. You need to eat or drink something that is quickly digested and turned into blood sugar. Orange juice or regular (nondiet) sodas are ideal. When you don't have access to something like that, you have to improvise—which is why we recommend you always have food or glucose tablets with you, everywhere you go. Hard candy, cookies, crackers, or any food high in carbohydrate is best, but even potatoes will eventually work. It doesn't have to be sugar, and it doesn't have to be a liquid.

Most episodes of hypoglycemia are mild, and once your blood glucose has returned to normal, there are usually no aftereffects. If an episode occurs when you are alone or with your family, there is little emotional reaction because you all know what is happening. If your friends or coworkers see you refusing help, sweating, and shaking, they may have a different attitude toward you when the episode is over. Even though they continue to be sympathetic and understanding, your relationship changes. They are uneasy about what might happen the next time. If you are prepared for hypoglycemia with foods to eat and if you prepare your family, friends, coworkers, fellow students, teachers, and coaches, then they will know what to do to help you and a highly emotional event will be avoided for you all.

Hypoglycemia but Not Diabetes?

It is a rare event to have blood glucose drop below 60 mg/dl for people who do not have diabetes and are not taking medications to lower blood sugar. This can occur at times of prolonged fasting especially in women, and in starvation, and with alcoholism. Even more rarely, it can occur because of diseases such as adrenal or pituitary gland failure, or because of tumors that produce insulin or insulin-like hormones. (Insulin-producing tumors only occur in four cases per one million patient-years.) If blood glucose is below 60 mg/dl after an overnight fast of 12 hours and is accompanied by symptoms or signs of hypoglycemia (see chapter 1), then ask your doctor about a medical evaluation for potential causes of low blood glucose.

Reactive hypoglycemia is defined as low blood glucose occurring after meals or snacks containing high amounts of sugars. It can occur due to rapid emptying of the stomach following stomach surgery or for unknown causes. Reactive hypoglycemia typically occurs 30–90 minutes after a meal.

There are people who experience symptoms of anxiety, nervousness, hunger, tremor, nausea, and chest pain or tightness, which are very much like the adrenaline symptoms of hypoglycemia listed in Table 1-1. They may also experience some of the symptoms attributed to brain starvation like tiredness, confusion, weakness, mood changes, headache, and numbness or tingling around the mouth, nose, or tongue. Almost never do people who have reactive hypoglycemia develop signs of extremely low blood sugar such as paralysis, involuntary muscle contractions, seizures, unconsciousness, or coma.

It is normal for insulin levels to rise after consuming foods that are converted to glucose in the intestine and then absorbed, which raises blood sugar. A very small number of people seem to overproduce insulin, and they have below normal blood sugar levels as a result. There are individuals whose blood glucose drops to 40 mg/dl, but they still do not develop obvious symptoms. A rise in adrenaline levels, which helps to raise blood sugar, almost always causes the symptoms of reactive hypoglycemia when they occur. Eating small quantities of sugar-containing food usually relieves these symptoms.

The current medical opinion regarding diagnosis of reactive hypoglycemia is that people who experience these symptoms should test their blood glucose using a self-blood glucose-monitoring meter when they are having symptoms.

If blood sugar levels are consistently below 65 mg/dl, then they may have reactive hypoglycemia. They should consult their physician. There is no evidence that reactive hypoglycemia is a warning sign of impending diabetes.

If you have reactive hypoglycemia following stomach surgery, then eating 5–6 small meals instead of any large ones may reduce the symptoms. People who have rapid gastric emptying can benefit from medicines that slow down stomach emptying. Some people who eat a diet low in concentrated sweets are able to reduce the frequency and severity of symptoms. Many people with reactive hypoglycemia find that their symptoms go away over time.

Since the symptoms of hypoglycemia can be mimicked by emotional disturbances such as anxiety and depression, many scientific investigators speculate that disturbed brain chemistry accounts for the symptoms. This explanation is most reasonable when blood sugar below 65 mg/dl cannot be documented at the time symptoms occur. If emotional disturbances appear to be the cause, then the patient needs medication or counseling to relieve the symptoms.

2

The Risks of Highs and Lows

All people with diabetes who require insulin face a tough dilemma. Tight control of your blood glucose keeps you healthier, but it also increases your chances of going too low. Although these episodes can be unpleasant, may pose a safety risk, and sometimes are embarrassing, the real question is, how harmful are they? Is there sufficient research to compare the risks of poor control (which means you have too high blood sugar levels) with the risks of low blood sugar? How can you decide what levels of blood sugar control are reasonable? Reasonable means that you want to live a full, active life and avoid later serious complications of diabetes.

First the good news. There is strong research evidence that good control of blood glucose does help prevent the complications of diabetes. Some of you will claim that you know friends or relatives who are extremely sloppy in their control and yet don't seem to develop any complications. Others of you will claim that you know people who have been very careful of their blood sugar control but still developed early and severe complications. Yes, that sometimes happens, but both of these developments are exceptions. The research shows that this is not what happens to the majority of people. People who have poor diabetes control are more likely to develop the complications of diabetes.

The Benefits of Good Control

The long-awaited results of the Diabetes Control and Complications Trial (DCCT) were published in September 1993. This study began in 1983 and involved 1,441 people with insulin dependent diabetes; most of them were either free of or had minimal signs of complications. The average age was 27; half of the subjects were women. They had been randomly assigned to an intensive treatment group or to a conventional diabetes treatment group.

The study showed that tight control of blood glucose definitely reduced the frequency and severity of the complications of diabetes. Intensive diabetes management reduced the risk of kidney disease by 35% and of kidney failure by more than 50%. These patients reduced their risk of developing eye complications (retinopathy) by 76%. Their risk of nerve damage (neuropathy) was reduced by 60%. Because the findings were so dramatic, the study ended a year early so the results could be published and health care providers could use them in developing diabetes care strategies with their patients.

We also know that people who already have signs of complications can improve their condition by getting better blood glucose control. For example, ophthalmologists have photographed the reversal of damage in the retina of the eye after patients began intensive glucose control. And as you might expect, the reverse is true, too. The eye damage got rapidly worse when patients slipped into poor glucose control.

A large multi-year study of people with type 2 diabetes called the United Kingdom Prospective Diabetes Study

(UKPDS) found that maintaining near-to-normal blood glucose levels provided the same benefits and protection from complications for people with type 2.

Don't overlook the other benefits of maintaining as near to normal blood glucose levels as possible. You will feel better. Many people who consistently have blood glucose levels in the 200s or higher do not function well and complain of fatigue. They feel tired and cranky and sit around all day. They also have more infections, colds, and flu. Studies have shown that white blood cells defend against infections more effectively when the blood glucose is near normal. It makes sense that when your blood sugar is nearer normal, every process in your body will be nearer normal, too.

Now, improved control does not guarantee that you will be free of complications—there appears to be a genetic influence that we cannot control. But even if you have that genetic tendency, the odds are still in your favor if you achieve good blood glucose control. When you have diabetes, the biggest concerns for your health are heart disease, kidney failure, and stroke. You protect yourself against those conditions with good blood glucose control and controlling blood pressure and cholesterol. Occasional low blood sugar seems like a small price to pay for such valuable benefits.

The Risks of Good Control

We also learned from the DCCT that people in the intensive diabetes management group had more episodes of low blood glucose. If you keep your blood sugar closer to normal, it is easier to slip to the low side. There are potential risks associated with individual episodes of low blood glucose. For example, the risk of having an automobile accident while driving with low blood glucose is a great concern (chapter 13). The risks of other accidents both at home and at work are much greater if your blood glucose is low. But aside from accidents, is there damage to your body from an episode of low blood sugar?

We must distinguish between mild hypoglycemia and severe hypoglycemia. In the first, you may be shaky and disoriented, but conscious. While you may need assistance, you are likely to be able to drink juice on your own. With severe hypoglycemia, you are more likely to be nearly unconscious and must have assistance. During severe hypoglycemic episodes, you may have convulsions, which can cause some damage to muscles and bones. It is rare to find fractures of legs, upper arms, and shoulders. Compression fractures involving the vertebra in the upper back can also occur but are extremely rare. Muscular strains and sprains are more common. People usually find that they have muscle soreness the day after a severe nighttime low. This is caused by the strenuous contractions of muscle groups during the convulsive jerking of the body. Severe brain damage and death is a possibility when the hypoglycemia has been severe and lasted for many hours.

The long-range effects of one or two severe hypoglycemic episodes per year and several mild episodes per week are difficult to evaluate. We can measure the effect of low blood sugar on mental function while it is happening, but it is extremely difficult to measure the long-term effects. To do that we would need to start testing the moment the diabetes diagnosis was made and perform tests periodically over the lifetime of the patient, or at least over a period of many years. In addition, it is very difficult to determine how severe the episode was.

So, we turn to our own experience for information. It is reassuring that many people with insulin dependent diabetes have survived more than 40 years of diabetes, have had many mild and severe hypoglycemic episodes, and have still achieved recognition in intellectually demanding careers. Table 2-1 lists some of the famous people who have lived with diabetes and had full careers. Now, no one in his right mind would recommend that you take a cavalier attitude toward hypoglycemia. Severe hypoglycemia probably takes its toll on brain cells. Your goal is to treat hypoglycemia before it gets severe so you can limit severe episodes as much as possible and still maintain good diabetes control.

None of us have the personal discipline or the environment to control diet, exercise, and medication as we would in

TABLE 2-1

Famous People with Diabetes

Athletes
Sugar Ray Robinson, boxing
JoAnne Washham, pro golf
Bill Talbot, tennis
Ron Santos, Chicago Cubs, baseball
Corbin Mills, bike racing
Wade Wilson, Minnesota Vikings, football
Michael Treacy, ski jumping
Arthur Ashe, tennis
Ned Edwards, squash champion
Chuck Heidenreich, skiing
Kurt Fraser, Chicago Black Hawks, hockey

Entertainers
Giacomo Puccini, composer
Jackie Gleason, comedian
Elvis Presley, singer
Peggy Lee, singer
Mary Tyler Moore, actress
Minnie Pearl, comedienne
Otto Preminger, producer

World Leaders
Mikhail Gorbachev
Anwar Sadat

Business Executives
Howard Hughes
Ray Kroc (founder of McDonald's)

Politicians
Ralph Bunche, UN diplomat and Nobel Prize winner
Fiorello H. LaGuardia, former mayor of New York City

a diabetes ward of a large research hospital. However, to limit the number of severe lows you're going to experience, you need to learn to control food, exercise, and medication as best you can. We, the authors, have chosen to pursue a lifestyle that aims for good blood glucose control and accepts the risks of occasional episodes of hypoglycemia. We have lived with diabetes for more than 110 years between us and are relatively free of complications, even though we have had thousands of episodes of hypoglycemia. These are the positive results that we present to you.

3

Checking Your Levels

Your blood glucose meter is the best tool you have for fine-tuning your glucose levels and avoiding hypoglycemia. In fact, we're lucky to have glucose meters. This is the most important advance in the management of diabetes since the discovery of insulin. But many people don't use one. We'll discuss some of the excuses for why they don't later in this chapter, but the result is poor diabetes control and a huge problem with serious complications. So this chapter is dedicated to explaining how and why to monitor your blood glucose every day. We want to overcome all excuses for not doing it.

When you have diabetes, you always have to think about how your food intake, your exercise, and the amount of diabetes medication you've taken will influence your blood glucose level over the next few hours. Will any of the three cause you to have low blood glucose? The first step is to think, "What was my blood glucose level the last time I checked it, and what is it now? Do I need to check it again now? Are there any other factors that might be influencing my blood sugar, such as stress, fatigue, or illness?" When in doubt—and to avoid going too low—use your glucose meter.

Now, you may wonder why you can't use urine testing instead. For many years, that was the only way to measure blood sugar—to wait until it got high enough to spill over into the urine. The problem with using urine testing for glucose is that the results are not accurate or reliable. A study was done to compare urine and blood glucose samples collected as close together as possible in thousands of patients. In more than half the patients, the urine test indicated high levels of sugar (from 1+ to 4+) but the level of sugar in the blood was near normal. The only time for you to use urine testing is when you're checking for ketones.

How To Do It

Learning to use a blood glucose meter is relatively simple. Your provider or diabetes educator can teach you. And you can call the meter company for assistance any time. Most people benefit from having their educator or provider check their "metering technique" every year or so—especially if you're getting some odd results. This is a good time to find out if there have been any new developments in blood glucose monitoring, too.

To self-monitor blood glucose (SMBG), you need a drop of blood to put on the test strip or directly into the meter. You need to be sure that your hands are clean and completely dry, with no lotion or other substance to interfere with getting a good sample. You get the blood by puncturing the skin with a lancet (a spring-loaded tiny blade or laser). You put the drop of blood on the strip and insert it in the meter, or put the drop on the special pad in the meter. In less than a minute, you can read the glucose level on a digital readout.

Why You Do It

Our bodies do not give signals to our brain about blood sugar levels until sugar is dangerously high or low. You need to know what your blood glucose level is to make realistic adjustments in the food you eat and when you eat it, how much exercise to get and when, and in the amount of diabetes medication you plan to take and when you plan to take it. By checking your blood glucose at various times each day, usually before meals and at bedtime, you can begin to see the patterns of how food, exercise, and medication affect your blood glucose. You can learn when your particular type and dosage of insulin or oral medication has its greatest effect and when your blood glucose usually reaches its lowest point.

Many people have difficulty figuring out how to use the information in their blood glucose records. You may want your physician to just prescribe a schedule for you, so you don't have to think about it. However, it isn't that simple. You have your own lifestyle, and no doctor or educator can prescribe a treatment plan that will fit your varying schedule of eating and exercise. You must learn to do this for yourself with help from your diabetes educator or physician.

Ask yourself questions about the number you get when you check your blood glucose. When you get a high reading, ask "Why is my blood sugar so high? Did I eat too much at my last meal? Was it because I didn't go for my walk this morning? Was it because I slept in this morning and took my insulin two hours later than I usually do?" When your blood glucose is surprisingly low, you need to ask "Why is it so low? Did exercise bring it down? Did I eat less carbohydrate than usual?" This questioning process lasts only a moment or two but can be very helpful. Only by getting some understanding of the changes in your glucose level will you learn how to adjust your own insulin, eating, and exercise patterns. As you get more experience with it, your self-confidence will improve, and you can be more and more flexible in your lifestyle.

Why People Don't Do It

We have observed that patients have predicable problems or concerns about doing blood glucose monitoring—pain, support or help, time, cost, and confusion about how to use the results.

Pain. Getting the blood sample is very important. You use an automatic spring-loaded puncturing device that holds a sharp lancet or a laser lancet to obtain the drop of blood. People who haven't tried it fear that it is painful. The lancets are tiny and very sharp, so they produce little pain. The laser lancet has no blade and does not cause pain. Using the sides of the finger rather than the center makes for less soreness later. Some meters can use a blood sample from a site other than the fingers, such as the forearm, which is said to be painless. Talk with your doctor or educator about what works best for you.

Keep an eye out for new products because manufacturers are working hard to find painless, effective tools for you. The GlucoWatch is a new device that gives blood sugar readings without a finger prick. However, you still have to use your other meter to see whether the GlucoWatch results are accurate.

Help. Most people, even children younger than 10 years old, are capable of checking their own blood sugar. No one (except tiny children) should depend on another person to do his (her) blood glucose checks or use that as an excuse for not doing them. When you depend on someone else, you put unfair demands on that person, and you lose independence and the sense of responsibility for your own illness.

However, your family and friends should know how to check your blood sugar. In an emergency, they may need to check it because you cannot do it yourself.

Time. Although a glucose check usually requires less than three minutes to do, you may think that you just don't have time for it. These are probably the most valuable minutes you spend on yourself each day, no matter how busy you are.

It is necessary to occasionally recalibrate your meter in order for it to measure glucose correctly. Some people are annoyed at having to spend time to do this, but you need to be sure that you can trust the results of your glucose checks. Otherwise, what's the point of doing them? Follow the directions that come with the meter. Call the company for assistance, and when necessary, they can send a new test solution to check the results.

Cost. The cost of each glucose check may concern you. Meters are often discounted or sometimes even free in special promotions. However, if your meter uses strips, the strips can cost more than $0.60 each, so to do 4 checks a day would cost $2.40. Most medical insurance pays for the strips if you use insulin. If you take oral medications, you need to ask whether meters and strips are covered under your plan. You might try a meter that doesn't require strips. Discuss the different meters and which would work best for you with your diabetes educator. Others just don't do the glucose checks. The information you get from the blood glucose check is extremely valuable to you. When you consider the "cost" of diabetes complications, the meter and test strips are a good investment!

Confusion. Your blood glucose records may seem useless if you are collecting information only for your physician to interpret. Some people dutifully write the glucose check results in their logbook and then during their periodic medical visits, hand the book to their physician or diabetes educator. When they do this, sometimes it seems like they are saying, "Here is my record, tell me what it means. Tell me what to do." Some physicians and educators have encouraged patients to be passive like this. Their attitude seems to be, "I am the authority. I will tell you what to do. You must obey me. You are just a mere patient."

Even if you want this kind of relationship, it just won't work and ends up frustrating everyone—doctors, educators, and patients. Diabetes is different. It's not like a broken bone or pneumonia; it can't be cured. You have to take it everywhere you go, so you are the only one who can make decisions on the spot about what to do. A diabetes educator can help you learn how to use your blood checks to decide what to eat, how much medication to take, and how much exercise to get. That's part of you becoming the expert on your own diabetes.

What to Expect from Your Health Care Provider

Your diabetes care providers need to motivate you to maintain good glucose control while at the same time encouraging you to be flexible and independent. When you have good rapport, you consider your provider and diabetes educator as teachers and friends. They are sharing their expertise with you so you can use it for your own challenges. If you, however, look at your provider as an authority figure who demands respect and obedience, it's not likely that you have a good relationship or that you are learning what you need to know to handle your own diabetes.

You should be comfortable describing the difficulties you are having and honest about your likes and dislikes. Don't agree to try something if you know that you just won't do it. You should feel that you are going to learn something at every visit, even when your diabetes is in good control.

Your physician is responsible for helping you manage your diabetes and needs to be sure that you know the many details about checking blood glucose, injecting insulin, and planning your meals. In many medical centers, much of this training is the responsibility of a team of diabetes educators who are often nurses or dietitians. Proper training is very important. When you have a life change, such as going to college, getting pregnant, changing jobs, competing athletically at a higher level, or retiring, you need to see an educator to help you make the necessary adjustments to the big three: food, exercise, and medication.

One of the most severe limitations for physicians and educators is time. Time is money, and most of them are under pressure to see many patients each day. Developing rapport takes time. Some busy health care providers have a tendency to recommend mathematical formulas that you can use in adjusting your insulin dosages to your glucose levels. These formulas are sometimes useful, but they are not a substitute for understanding how to think through each problem and solve it yourself. Much of this problem solving is accomplished through trial and error rather than by arithmetic. Using your own experience with the guidance of teachers is the best way to learn.

To sum up:

■ Develop an honest relationship.

■ Don't shirk your duties and responsibilities.

- Don't let them take your role away from you.

- Use their expertise.

- Use your experience.

What to Expect from Your Meter

Home glucose meters are accurate enough to help you control your diabetes, even though the results may vary more than 20% from the lab or "correct" result. That may not seem very accurate, but for the management of your diabetes, plus or minus 20% is still very useful. Your meter needs to be calibrated frequently to make sure it is working correctly. Many people find this irritating and time consuming and don't do it. A meter is like any other good piece of machinery: the results you get are as good as the care you take of it. With modern meters, the test result should be within 15% of the correct result when you do a calibration check. If it's not, ask your educator for help or call the meter manufacturer for advice.

Inaccurate results usually happen when the person using the meter makes mistakes. Basic problems include how you get the blood sample and put it on the strip or into the meter. In most meters, timing is automatic, but it can be a problem in some of the older meters. Defective strips are always a possibility, but most manufacturers have excellent quality control. If the strips are out-of-date or improperly stored, they may not give accurate results.

Frustration with the Numbers

Try not to get frustrated with blood sugar numbers you can't explain. Nobody has all the answers. So don't let individual results get you down; the number to focus on is your three-month average—your HbA1c. It's the one that tells you how you're really doing for the long term (see chapter 4).

The more you learn about your body, the more you know about things that can affect your blood sugar level. For example, a blood glucose reading can be strongly influenced by low red blood cell counts (anemia) or an excess of red cells (polycythemia). Anemia gives falsely high blood glucose readings, and polycythemia gives falsely low readings. Routine blood counts are recommended at least once a year so you'll know about chronic changes in blood cell levels.

Even if you have to guess what is causing the high or low blood glucose, make adjustments for it, and move on. Don't let it get you down or cause you to skip glucose checks the next day.

The Future of SMBG

Researchers are working on a glucose sensor that can be implanted underneath the skin that will determine the glucose level and show it on a meter worn like a wristwatch. Someday such information may be transmitted to a device that would automatically release an amount of rapid-acting insulin from an implanted insulin supply. It would be like an artificial pancreas. There would, however, still be the problem of avoiding hypoglycemia. Rapid-acting insulin is now available, and people who use it report fewer episodes of hypoglycemia, because they are better able to time their insulin action with the rise in blood glucose from a meal.

The Bottom Line

The blood sugar checks that you do several times every day work like glasses for severely nearsighted people. Without glasses, these people are helpless because they can't see. Without frequent blood glucose checks, you can't see where you are and don't know where you are going. You don't know if you are high or low, so you don't know how much insulin you need to take or how much food you need to eat. With frequent blood glucose checks and some experience, you can improve the management of your own diabetes.

4

Your Batting Average

D o you know what the hemoglobin A1c test is? You may be getting one several times a year but don't know what it's telling you. Many people don't understand, and some busy physicians only have time to say, "It's too high, and we need to get it lower." If you understand what it is, you can use it to improve your health.

Simply put, the HbA1c test measures your blood sugar "batting average" over the past 2–3 months. For example, during one game, a baseball player may have 3 hits out of 5 times at bat for an average for that game of .600. What really counts, however, is what the player's average is at the end of the season—after many games. Any player who hits .300 for a season is an outstanding hitter. The glycohemoglobin test is like a batting average for the season because it measures your average blood glucose over the last 3 months.

What's in a Name?

Let's look at each part of the name of this important blood test—HbA1c. Hemoglobin (Hb) is the red protein in red blood cells that carries oxygen from the lungs to all the tissues in the body. While it does this job, hemoglobin also picks up glucose in nearly the same proportion that it exists in your blood. The sugar coats the hemoglobin, so it becomes a special kind of glycated (glucose-coated) hemoglobin called A1c.

Red cells are being formed in the bone marrow at the same rate as they are dying—about a million a second. Their life span is 60–90 days. At any one moment, a sample of your blood contains a mixture of red blood cells of all ages from brand new to about 3 months old. The coating process is slow and once the hemoglobin has a coating, it does not give it up even if the blood glucose level gets very low. The glycated hemoglobin remains in the red blood cells until they die and are removed from the circulation.

What's My Goal?

The goal of diabetes control is to try to keep the A1c test as near normal (4–6%) as possible. Unfortunately, studies have shown that people with insulin dependent diabetes who have lower A1c levels have a higher number of both mild and severe hypoglycemic episodes than people with higher A1c levels. Generally speaking, the tighter you control your glucose, the greater the risk of hypoglycemia. But that doesn't mean you have to have more lows. Many people accomplish near-normal A1c levels without having more episodes of severely low blood sugar.

Together with your physician and diabetes educator choose an HbA1c level that suits your health goals and situation. Young children, people who don't have warning signs of hypoglycemia, and people with frequent nighttime lows or many episodes of severe hypoglycemia may need to have higher goals than the ideal of 6–7%. Otherwise, most physicians and laboratories interpret an HbA1c level higher than 8% as an indication of poor glucose control. Values of 12–15% show extremely poor control, with blood glucose levels between 300 and 400 mg/dl over much of the last 3 months. (See Table 4-1.)

You should have an HbA1c test several times a year. People using insulin should have it checked four times a year. For people with type 2 diabetes using meal planning, exercise, and perhaps, diabetes pills, it needs to be checked at least twice a year, or more often if you are having difficulty achieving your target levels.

It is a number that you should know. Ask your physician to tell you your test result each time and put it in your record book, so you can see how you are doing from season to season. Your daily blood glucose checks give you one piece of important information, and the HbA1c gives you the other.

The HbA1c test is an extremely useful measure of how well you are controlling your blood glucose levels. It shows you how well you are doing over the long term. It is a good indication of how well you are doing at preventing complications, too. Many researchers believe that other cells in the body also get coated with glucose and that may lead to some of the complications of diabetes, such as nerve damage or poor circulation. When you keep blood glucose levels lower, then there is less coating of other cells.

The Highs and Lows

When you are watching your HbA1c for improvement, it's important to remember that it is a slow process. Once the hemoglobin has a coating, it keeps it. For example, if you have been under good control and you develop the flu or bronchitis, your glucose rises to high levels for days to maybe a

TABLE 4-1

Glucose Level and Fasting HbA1c Average

Blood Glucose (mg/dl)	HbA1c (%)
360	14
330	13
300	12
270	11
240	10
210	9
180	8
150	7
120	6
80	5

week or two. After a couple of weeks, everything gets back under good control. But, the amount of glycated hemoglobin went up during your sickness and will remain elevated for several months. Don't be discouraged because it will take more than a few weeks of good control to offset the effects of several weeks of poor control. When you make changes in your meal plan, exercise, and medication, don't expect your HbA1c test to improve rapidly. It will gradually respond to your efforts.

Then you may ask, "How come my HbA1c test is usually really good (6–7%) when I know that I have fairly frequent peaks of high blood glucose?" Here is where the concept of "average" is critical. If high peaks of glucose last only for a short time, for example for only a couple of hours, the hemoglobin does not get coated very much. Remember, it is a slow process. If an individual has low blood glucose levels frequently, there is much less coating than normal. Even when averaged with the few high peaks, the result may still be a normal HbA1c test level. When the test is high, such as 10–13%, it means that the blood glucose levels have been far above normal much of the time during the past 2 to 3 months.

Other things to consider

If you have a disease that affects the formation of red blood cells and hemoglobin, your provider must take great care in interpreting your HbA1c. Any disease that shortens the life span of a red blood cell will reduce the time it is exposed to glucose and decrease the A1c level. An iron deficiency anemia, however, may increase your A1c level, but it is not clear why. If you have arthritis and take large amounts of aspirin, your A1c level may be too high when it is measured by certain techniques. So, be sure to discuss other health conditions with your health care provider if you think they may be affecting your HbA1c.

All in all

People often don't understand why the A1c test level is a long-range average. If your control has been exceptionally good for a week, why doesn't that promptly improve the A1c level? It does improve it but not by much. In baseball, if a batter has a sensational hitting streak for only one week, his batting average at the end of the season does not improve much. It's getting hits at each game that improves it.

You may complain that to maintain tight control of your blood sugar you have to follow a rigid meal plan, exercise, and medication schedule just like you were in the hospital. You might feel that such tight control and your busy life just won't work together. Actually, by frequently checking your blood sugar and making adjustments, you can make your busy life run more smoothly, and you'll feel better, too. And by checking your blood glucose levels daily, you will avoid going too low by eating or adjusting your medication or exercise. Now you have the keys to good health with diabetes—please be sure to use them.

5

Treating Low Blood Sugar at Home

Treating low blood sugar at home should be simple. You just need to eat or drink something with carbohydrate in it. As the food is digested and absorbed, your blood glucose level rises. However, when the level falls too low, you may not be able to feed yourself. You may resist eating and have difficulty chewing or swallowing. You may fight being helped, have convulsions, or lapse into unconsciousness. To treat hypoglycemia always have food or beverages with you that are easy to swallow and are absorbed quickly.

Across the U.S. each year, ambulances make hundreds, even thousands, of trips to homes to take care of uncooperative, convulsing, or even unconscious people with severe hypoglycemia. Family members tend to panic when you are unable to eat. Their first impulse may be to run to the telephone and call for an ambulance. Frequently, the ambulance doesn't arrive for 15 minutes or longer, further delaying the treatment that you need. With a little training and a little confidence, your family members can handle most of the severe lows that occur at home.

Dr. Lincoln has lived with type 1 diabetes for more than 63 years. Only once did he have to be taken to the hospital in an ambulance for hypoglycemia. He was in an airport and collapsed in a hallway. People there thought he was having a heart attack (see chapter 14). His wife has been able to treat all his severe low blood sugars that have happened at home. Dr. Eaddy has survived 49 years with type 1 diabetes and only once had to be taken to the hospital in an ambulance. That episode occurred before glucagon was available to use at home.

The need to eat comes on slowly, but recognizing the need can be a major problem. When you have had diabetes for only a few years, you usually have early symptoms of falling blood sugar and have time to eat. Even so, people may fail to eat, get more confused, and no longer realize what they need to do. After 10–20 years with diabetes, you can lose the early symptoms of hypoglycemia (chapter 19), so how do you know when your glucose is falling? Frequent blood glucose checks will do it. You need to correct low blood glucose as quickly as possible, so don't delay if you check and it is low.

Treating Mild Hypoglycemia

You have probably developed a way that you like to treat low blood sugar—once you have figured out that it is low. All of us can describe times when we thought we were going low, but when we checked, our blood glucose was normal or even high. Other times we may have just been doing a routine check before a meal and found, to our surprise, that we were extremely low. You just can't guess what your blood glucose level is.

When you are away from home, however, you may not be able to check it. In those cases, eat a small amount of hard candy or drink half a can of regular soda to be safe. If you find that you did not need to eat, you can get your blood glucose back under control at the next meal.

What do you eat or drink?

For years, people have assumed that sugars are more rapidly digested than other carbohydrates. But research has shown that carbohydrates such as rice, bread, and potatoes have the same blood glucose effect as sugar. Obviously, you can't carry a bowl of rice or potatoes with you, and they take time to chew and to be absorbed. Liquid carbohydrates, such as orange juice or milk, avoid the chewing and time problem, but you need a way to carry them. When you are going low, it is important to eat or drink something that contains carbohydrate—crackers, bread, pudding, or whatever you can find. Foods that are high in fat, such as meat or chocolate, take longer to digest and be absorbed, so we don't recommend you use them.

Some treatment choices for mild to moderate hypoglycemia are listed in Table 5-1. There is no magic in the amounts given. The servings provide about 100 calories and enough carbohydrate to raise your blood glucose level.

Which food do you want to use?

Where you are when your blood sugar falls makes a big difference. Treatment at home usually is different from when you are at walking or at work or school. How convenient is the food to carry in your pocket or purse during the winter or summer? You need a food that is easy to unwrap, does not require a lot of chewing or sucking, is not in a heavy container,

TABLE 5-1

Foods to Treat Mild Hypoglycemia

Type of Food	Amount
Sweetened soda	6 oz
Fruit juices	1 cup
Raisins	2 Tbsp
Table sugar	2–3 Tbsp
Hard or soft candy	20–30 grams
Gumdrops	10
LifeSavers	5–7
Jelly beans	6
Honey or corn syrup	2 Tbsp
Cake frosting	1 tube (6.8 oz)
Chocolate cookies	2
M&Ms	25
Glucose tablets	2–5
Any carbohydrate	15–20 grams

is cheap, and is easy to get in any deli, drugstore, or grocery store. Let's look at some of the foods you might choose.

Sweetened sodas are ideal because they are absorbed quickly. But they cannot be easily carried with you. You may think, "ah, but there are always soda machines around." But they are not always where you need them to be. Or they may only be taking change not dollar bills—and you have no change. What if you are driving in the country and need a soda? You have to assume that everything can go wrong and plan ahead so you have what you need when you need it.

Fruit juices are highly effective in raising blood sugar quickly. They may be heavy to carry in pocket or purse, but are great for nighttime lows. Dr. Lincoln finds that grape and apple juice keep him awake if he has to drink some during the night. For him, orange juice works best. Canned juices have to be opened, or the straw must be inserted in boxes of juice. If you're too low, you may have trouble doing this. It can be a long trip from your bedroom to the kitchen to get a glass of juice. If you could have small bottles of juice with easy opening caps in your bedroom or a nearby bathroom, that would be ideal.

Raisins are easy to carry and often come in handy little boxes. They are soft and easy to chew and get the carbohydrate into your system pretty quickly.

Sugar cubes are good, but they crumble easily and spread in your purse or pocket. Even in a plastic baggie, they crumble and may be difficult to get into your mouth.

LifeSavers or hard candies are good, but the package has to be opened and if you've waited too long, that may be a problem. LifeSavers can be sucked but it takes a little time for them to be absorbed. If your blood glucose is really low, you need to be concerned about choking.

Soft non-chocolate candies work well but need to be carried in small plastic bags because they break easily.

Honey or corn syrup can be carried in a plastic bottle with a hole in the tip covered with a small cap. You can put the tip of the bottle in your mouth and squeeze. You have to swallow to digest the glucose.

Cake frosting comes ready made and packaged in tubes for ease of carrying.

Chocolate candy bars or cookies are fine but slow. The high-fat content slows down absorption of the carbohydrate in them. They can quickly become messy in your pocket or purse, especially in the summer.

M&M chocolate candies work well because they can be carried in a small plastic bag and don't melt easily. Each candy has about 4 calories. They're easy to chew and swallow. You can keep a large bag at home and refill the smaller bags as needed. Although the chocolate is rich in fat, the sugar coating is quickly converted to glucose.

Glucose tablets, gels, or liquid are flavored corn syrup or glucose solutions that are absorbed like sugar cubes are. The glucose products are more expensive but are conveniently packaged and you're not likely to eat too much. You open a tube of glucose gel and squeeze it into a corner of your mouth. In fact, others can put it between your cheek and gums if you're going too low, but you must swallow to be able to absorb the glucose. These can take 10–20 minutes to affect your blood glucose levels.

Other carbohydrate foods that contain a lot of fat or protein take much longer to digest and convert to glucose. This is why a chocolate candy bar or a cup of whole milk are not the best choice for treating low blood sugar.

Other factors

Most of us have had an experience where we have had hypoglycemia after we have started to eat a regular meal. The meal was not digested and absorbed fast enough to counteract the rapidly falling blood glucose. Some people have developed nerve damage that slows the emptying of their stomachs, and they need to use liquids to treat hypoglycemia if possible.

To each his own

Sooner or later, you and your family will develop ways to treat low blood sugar that work for you. There are hundreds of little tricks that people have developed to meet their special needs, and you will develop yours. The important thing is to eat or drink some form of rapidly absorbed carbohydrate food.

Watch for the rebound

A common question is "How much should I eat?" When you have mild hypoglycemia, you are usually hungry and uncomfortable. In fact, you want to keep eating until the symptoms go away. You have to remember that it takes 10–20 minutes to convert what you have eaten into blood glucose. So, stop eating to let that happen. If you eat until the symptoms disappear, you will eat much more than you need. The only exception is when you have been exercising vigorously and get low—it is usually wise to eat more than you usually do because exercise continues to lower your blood glucose for hours. See Table 5-2 for suggestions about how much carbohydrate to eat.

Try to remember the rule of 15-15. Take 15 grams of carbohydrate and wait 15 minutes. Check your blood sugar level, and eat another 15 grams if your level is still too low. When your blood sugar is coming back up, eat a protein and carbohydrate snack, such as half a meat sandwich or peanut butter crackers, to keep it in the normal ranges.

TABLE 5-2

How Much to Eat?

Blood glucose level (mg/dl)	Carbohydrate (g)
Under 40	30
40–50	25
51–60	20
61–80	15
80+ with symptoms	5–10

If you eat too much, you cause your blood sugar to re-bound too high. Then you need to bring that high glucose down. If you use diabetes medication to do it, please be careful and learn how to do it from your doctor or diabetes educator. It takes practice to do it safely (chapter 6). Your goal is to get your blood glucose levels down to normal in 2–4 hours. Rapid-acting insulin is ideal because it is absorbed quickly and will bring the blood glucose down in 1–2 hours. You have to be careful not to overshoot the mark or your blood sugar will be too low again. This is a cycle that you don't want to get into.

After you recover from mild to moderate hypoglycemia, you should be able to continue working or playing. After severe hypoglycemia, you may have muscle soreness, aching, and fatigue that lasts for a few hours. Sometimes there is some mild memory loss that lasts for a few hours. There is little reason to keep a child home from school the next day or not to go to work. Teachers, supervisors, and sometimes patients themselves have the idea that they have been damaged and need a day to recover. That is almost never the case. The sooner you get back to your normal life, the better you will feel.

Treating Severe Low Blood Sugar

When you cannot (or will not) eat because of severe hypoglycemia, you need to have glucagon available and a family member who can inject it. This will almost always prevent the need to call an ambulance. Everyone in the household should know how to prepare and inject glucagon. It is simple to do after a little practice. Family members need to read the instructions carefully and practice what to do if you have a severe hypoglycemic attack. If the box of glucagon is just put in the medicine cabinet and no one practices using it, your family members will probably not be able to react in a time of crisis. It is difficult to read the instructions in the glucagon package when a loved one is convulsing or is becoming unconscious. Family members have to be ready to act. Being uncertain or unsure of what they need to do means that they cannot take prompt action to help you.

Your doctor must write you a prescription for glucagon, and you must check the expiration date and get a new prescription when it goes out of date. You and your doctor should explain to your family that what you say or do during severe hypoglycemia is frequently not rational. You may resist treatment, become obnoxious, or even try to hit them, but you are not aware of what you are saying or doing. The higher centers of your brain are not functioning properly. Often you will not even remember what you did or said during a low. Whoever gives you the glucagon has to be firm but reassuring. If your helper becomes angry, this often causes you to resist more forcefully. You protest, "I'm all right. I don't need to eat. Leave me alone. Go away." But your helper has to keep trying and saying calm words like "Once you calm down, we will check your glucose and you can take some more insulin if necessary. For now, please do it for my sake. Please let me help you." This may have to be repeated calmly and firmly many times.

Once the glucagon solution is prepared (which takes about a minute), it can be injected wherever there is skin with a little fat under it. Good places are the abdomen, buttocks, upper arms, or thighs. If you are resisting, your helper may need more help to hold you down for the few seconds it takes to give the injection. It is injected under the skin but not into the muscle. If possible, massage the injection site for a minute or two to speed absorption of the glucagon.

After glucagon has been prepared for injection, it cannot be stored. It must be used immediately or thrown away. You may not want to go through the steps of preparing the glucagon for injection if you're just practicing and you'll have to throw it away. But in a future emergency, practice can be of great value—to you.

The instructions for giving glucagon are on the package. This sentence is printed in red at the top of the page of instructions enclosed in the box, "Become familiar with the following instructions before the emergency arises." A severe low blood sugar emergency may not occur for many months after you purchase the glucagon. Your initial training is easy to forget. Just like you have fire drills at school or at work, you and your family, friends, or coworkers need to rehearse and periodically review exactly what you will do when an emergency arises. This is how you avoid confusion and panic. And get your needs taken care of quickly.

Deciding when to use glucagon

If you can drink sweetened cola or fruit juice or chew a glucose tablet, then you don't need glucagon. If you are convulsing, are semi-conscious or unconscious, or are completely uncooperative, then you need to be given glucagon. Be sure that your family, friends, and coworkers understand when you need help and how to help you.

When a person consumes alcoholic beverages, glucose release from the liver is reduced. The glucagon injection will not work as well. If the person who has been drinking is unconscious or convulsing, it is safest to call an ambulance. He may need intravenous (IV) glucose (chapter 15).

Table 5-3 shows treatments that others can choose to help you with severely low blood sugar. Again, if you are not conscious or able to swallow, glucagon is the choice.

What do you do then?

As soon as you wake up and are able to swallow, you need something to eat. Glucagon alone is not sufficient. It provides a temporary rise in blood glucose. You need to drink additional sweet liquids or eat sweet foods. Because glucagon can cause you to become nauseated, be sure to tell your helpers to turn your head to the side in case vomiting occurs. Nausea after the administration of glucagon is common. When it does

TABLE 5-3

Treatments for Severe Hypoglycemia

1. Glucagon
2. Regular sodas (not diet)
3. Fruit juices
4. Glucose and sucrose tablets, gels, or liquids
5. Honey, corn syrup, or cake frosting

occur, after the nausea and vomiting are over, which is usually in a short time, you need to drink sweetened liquids. If possible, you should be sitting up when you eat or drink to avoid choking.

What to expect

The first time a family member gives a glucagon injection, she may expect an immediate response. It usually takes about 10 minutes before signs of recovery appear. Anxiety runs high in family members. It is often during these minutes of waiting that some member of the family can't stand the uncertainty and will call an ambulance. By the time the ambulance arrives, the patient is almost always awake and is often eating, too.

If you do not come around in 15 minutes, you should be given a second dose of glucagon, and your blood sugar level needs to be checked. This is the time that your family and friends need to know how to use your monitor! You may wake up before your blood glucose has started to rise. It usually takes 10 minutes before the glucose rises even 20 mg/dl. If your helper finds that your blood glucose is above 60 mg/dl, and you don't show any signs of waking up, then some other medical emergency may be happening. Unconsciousness has causes other than hypoglycemia. In such cases, call the ambulance immediately.

6

Adjusting Your Insulin to Avoid Hypoglycemia

This chapter offers advice about how to adjust your insulin dose to control your blood glucose better. Before you attempt to make any changes to the treatment plan you already have, discuss your ideas and what you want to change with your doctor and diabetes educator. Ask them for help and for more information about how to improve your blood glucose control.

Each of us responds differently to insulin, exercise, food, stress, and illness. The suggestions offered in this book are meant to stimulate your thinking about how you can manage your diabetes better and keep down the number of times that you have low blood sugar. Until you have had a lot of experience in making small adjustments in your insulin dose, be cautious. When you adjust your insulin dose, try to keep the other factors that affect your blood sugar as steady as possible. This means that you need to manage your meal plan, exercise, and stress to prevent major changes in them at the same time that you are adjusting the dose. Your records of how much your blood glucose changes when you change your insulin dose will tell you what works for you.

Since the discovery of insulin, a great deal has been discovered about how it works. There are many types of insulin. Human insulin (made in a laboratory with recombinant DNA technology) acts faster and has a shorter duration than animal insulin. Human insulin is more effective in preventing high blood glucose levels after meals.

Table 6-1 describes the types of insulin and the usual time of action of each one. The earlier onset of action, peak of action, and shorter duration of action for human insulin makes it appealing to you as you try to improve your blood sugar control. These are average times.

Unfortunately, with each injection, there is a variation in the absorption rate. You need to know what speeds up or slows down the rate at which your insulin goes to work, so you can get steady results.

TABLE 6-1

Insulin Action Time

Insulin Type	Onset	Peak (hours)	Duration (hours)
Human			
Lispro	5–15 min	30–90 min	4–6
Regular	30–60 min	2–3	3–6
NPH	2–4 hr	4–10	10–16
Lente	3–4 hr	4–12	12–18
Ultralente	6–10 hr	—	18–20
Insulin glargine	1.1 hr	—	24
Animal			
Regular	.5–2 hr	3–4	4–6
NPH	4–6 hr	8–14	16–20
Lente	4–6 hr	8–14	16–20

What causes insulin action to vary?

Dr. Eaddy says, "I hate to have hypoglycemia at night when I'm asleep. My bed gets wet with sweat. My wife wakes up and can't get back to sleep. When I drag myself to the refrigerator, I can't stop eating until my symptoms of low blood sugar go away. I have then eaten at least three times as much food as necessary to raise my blood glucose to a safe level. Then I am cold and find it unpleasant to crawl back into my wet bed. The next morning my blood glucose level might be over 300. I feel bad!

I rarely have nighttime lows, but I had four in one month. Why? The answer came by looking for changes in my daily routine. I had recently bought a hot tub. I discovered that when I took my bedtime shot of insulin and used the hot tub to relax before going to bed, I went low in the middle of the night. When I took the bedtime insulin after the hot tub dip, no problem!" Local heat is just one of the variables that affect how fast insulin is absorbed (Table 6-2). This effect is most easily seen when you inject rapid-acting or short-acting insulin.

As Table 6-2 shows, the things that affect how fast or how well the insulin is absorbed are local heat, environmental temperature, exercise, site and depth of the injection, type of insulin, and what mixture of insulin you use.

Local heat over an injection site shortly after the injection speeds up absorption of the insulin. You get the same effect if the site is vigorously massaged for several minutes until the skin becomes red and warm.

Warm room air or being immersed in warm water can dramatically increase the insulin absorption rate. One study

TABLE 6-2

Factors that Affect Insulin Absorption

- Local heat
- Environmental temperature
- Exercise
- Site of injection
- Depth of injection
- Type of insulin
- Insulin mixture

showed a 3 to 5 times higher absorption rate and significantly lower blood glucose after breakfast when air temperature was 86°F compared to 50°F.

Exercise combined with warm air stimulates insulin absorption. You may need to make adjustments in your meal plan or insulin dose to avoid hypoglycemia after exercising in warm temperatures. There are no rigid guidelines for how much of an adjustment you should make. Some suggestions are given later in this chapter. Careful observation and keeping records of your trial and error attempts will help you make adjustments in the future to your meal plan or insulin dose.

Exercise combined with injection in a limb increases absorption rate when the arm or leg is vigorously used. To control this variable, inject into a non-exercising part, such as the abdomen. Because exercise and insulin both lower blood sugar, when you exercise, you should consider adjustments to your food intake and insulin dose.

The site of the injection affects how fast the insulin is absorbed. For years, we were taught to rotate injection sites among legs, arms, buttocks, and abdominal areas. Recent studies show that this practice makes insulin action erratic and results in poor glucose control. If you use abdominal sites with regular insulin, you get lower peak blood sugar levels after meals than when you inject into your thigh. The time required for insulin to reach its peak concentration is much shorter from an abdominal injection than from the arm, thigh, or buttocks.

To be able to predict what the insulin will do and when it will do it, use only your abdomen for injection sites. Rotate the site over the abdomen, avoiding the middle around the navel where the blood supply is not as good. Use sites from just below the rib cage to just above the groin and pubic region. Don't develop the habit of selecting just one or two small areas. Repeated injections may cause local build-up of fat, which can decrease the absorption rate.

Occasionally a small blood vessel may be nicked during an injection. Bleeding from the puncture site may occur or a bruise may form. Although this may be an unpleasant sight, it is not a cause for concern. Insulin absorption is not usually affected, and you are not more likely to have low blood sugar.

Depth of injection is important. Insulin is absorbed most evenly when it is injected into the layer of fat just beneath the skin. When you inject more deeply into muscle, the rate of absorption is usually faster. When you inject into the skin, the absorption is more unpredictable than if you inject into fat. With the syringes currently available, the needle should be inserted perpendicular to the surface of the skin. If you are very thin with minimal fat underneath the skin, insert the needle at an angle of 45° to the skin.

Insulin of different types will be absorbed at different rates. Synthetic human insulin is absorbed more quickly and has a shorter duration of action than animal insulin. To control your blood sugar you need to know how to time your injections to work with meals and exercise. Rapid-acting synthetic human insulin is especially useful for busy people who may have to make frequent adjustments to their insulin schedule. Take note when you first use rapid-acting insulin before a meal, and you exercise within 60–90 minutes of the meal. Your blood sugar may fall more rapidly than you expect. Keep a record of what happens for a few times, and then you can adjust your eating and exercising times to fit your particular schedule.

It is now clear that rapid-acting insulin causes fewer episodes of nighttime lows, especially during sleep. For some reason, when your blood glucose starts getting low, you are much more likely to wake up. If you have had severe hypoglycemia during the night and you have been taking regular insulin before the evening meal, you may want to switch to rapid-acting insulin.

An advantage of rapid-acting human insulin is that it works quickly to bring the rise of blood sugar down after a meal and then it goes away. Regular insulin usually acts on the body longer than that. So, if you take rapid-acting insulin, you'll probably also need a small amount of long-acting insulin (NPH, ultralente, or glargine) at bedtime to prevent blood glucose rising at other times of the day.

When you change the type of insulin you use, it is important to carefully monitor your blood glucose at each meal and at bedtime, so you can see the different effects the new insulin is having. You need to be sure that you understand how the new insulin works. Ask questions of your physician until you feel comfortable with the change. Show your blood glucose records to your doctor or educator so you can work together on getting the most benefits from the new insulin. For example, you take rapid-acting insulin right before you eat. But, if your blood glucose is below 70 mg/dl, you might start the meal with fruit juice to bring your blood glucose up. Or you might eat and then take your insulin. You need to develop your game plan for how best to use the action time of your insulin.

We have found rapid-acting insulin to be a valuable tool in controlling our blood glucose levels. We look forward to new developments in insulin, such as glargine, a peakless long-acting insulin, which has just come on the market.

Using a mixture of insulin may or may not affect the speed of action or absorption. Rapid-acting human insulin can be mixed in the syringe with ultralente and NPH without changing the insulin effects. Regular and NPH insulin may be mixed in the same syringe or bottle without changing the time of action of either insulin. However, when regular is mixed with either lente or ultralente insulin, you may get a delay in the absorption of regular insulin. Insulin glargine cannot be mixed with other insulin. Pre-mixed insulin is convenient but may reduce your ability to fine-tune your control.

The effects of illness

Illness can affect insulin action and blood sugar control. Infections usually increase your need for insulin. Even seemingly minor infections such as gum disease or skin sores can make a difference. Obesity can greatly increase insulin requirements, as can pregnancy. Hormone diseases, such as hypothyroidism (decreased thyroid hormone production) or Cushing's syndrome (increased adrenal cortical hormone) may lead to difficulty maintaining good blood sugar control. Hyperthyroidism (increased thyroid hormone production) and chronic kidney failure can be a cause of unexpected low blood sugars. Some cancers produce hormone-like substances that act like insulin and cause low blood sugar. Discuss any unexplained increase or decrease in your insulin needs with your doctor. This is another good reason to have an annual physical exam.

Choosing Your Insulin Plan

When you and your doctor decide which types of insulin you should use, you are trying to mimic the action of a healthy pancreas. Figure 6-1 shows the insulin and glucose levels of a person who does not have diabetes. Very small amounts of insulin are required to keep blood glucose at a low normal level between midnight and breakfast time. As soon as breakfast is eaten, blood sugar rises and so does insulin concentration in the blood. At each meal or snack, blood glucose rises and so does insulin. It is this immediate release of insulin from the healthy pancreas that maintains normal blood glucose levels. If the person eats a large amount of carbohydrate foods, the pancreas releases insulin to cover it.

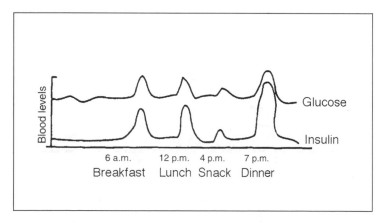

FIGURE 6-1 Typical changes in glucose and insulin levels over 24 hours in someone without diabetes.

When you eat a larger than usual amount of carbohydrate, your fixed dose of insulin may not be enough to bring the rise in blood glucose down. You must understand the process so that you can adjust your meal and your insulin to keep your blood sugar within normal levels.

Figures 6-2 and 6-3 show how different combinations of insulin work. The plan in Figure 6-2 would meet the needs of a busy person who gets up at the same time each day and eats three meals at about the same times each day. If you want a bedtime snack, then a small dose of rapid-acting insulin can be mixed with the bedtime dose of NPH.

As we see in Figure 6-3, doses of rapid-acting or short-acting insulin before each meal reduce the after-meal rise of blood glucose. Since you time the insulin injection to the meal, you can be more flexible about when you eat in your daily schedule. The action of rapid-acting and short-acting insulin is more predictable than intermediate-acting or long-acting insulin.

There are many ways to mix insulin effects to match your daily schedule. Ask your doctor for help.

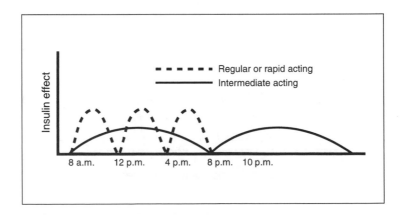

FIGURE 6-2 Split and mixed regular and intermediate insulin in two shots.

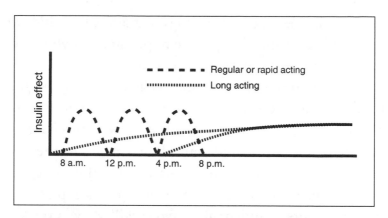

FIGURE 6-3 Three shots: split and mixed morning dose, regular dose, split and mixed evening dose.

Should you adjust your own insulin dose?

You and your physician should decide whether it is safe for you to adjust your own dose of insulin. The issues to consider that determine whether you are ready are listed in Table 6-3.

TABLE 6-3

ARE YOU READY TO CHANGE YOUR INSULIN DOSE?

Eaddy's Law tells you what to think about:

E   Exercise frequency and intensity

A   Ability to keep good records

D   Desire and ability to adjust your insulin dose

D   Diabetic complications

Y   Your ability to do 3 or 4 glucose checks a day

L   Lifestyle

A   Ability to detect early symptoms

W   Willingness to adjust your meal plan

If you have learned about the things that affect how and when insulin works and are willing to be responsible for your decisions, then you are likely to be successful.

You will need teaching and then coaching as you begin, but with practice, you can become your own coach. The daily management of diabetes is like a game. To win, you have to want to play it well. You and your physician choose the target blood glucose goals. You learn the basic skills of playing and the rules of the game. Then you practice, practice, practice until you become confident about your skill. As you track your progress by examining your blood sugar score card, you cheer and give yourself a pat on the back every time you hit your goal or figure out a way to get back to it. If you get stuck, ask for help from your doctor or diabetes educator, dietitian, exercise consultant, or counselor. The best teams have more than one player, so don't try to do it all by yourself all the time.

7

Using Your Meal Plan to Control Your Blood Sugar

M any years ago when we were first diagnosed with diabetes, we were told we would have to take insulin and follow a strict diet for the rest of our lives. At that time, food portions were weighed or carefully measured, and we ate fixed amounts of meat, vegetables, fruits, and bread and milk products at each meal. Sugar was not allowed except for the treatment of "insulin reactions." Diet was the mainstay of the treatment of diabetes, and a rigid schedule of injections of insulin was prescribed to keep sugar in the urine as low as possible. At that time, the only way to measure blood glucose was with a laboratory test performed in a hospital or clinic.

Dr. Lincoln says: When I began treatment for my diabetes back in 1938, I recall vividly being advised to inject 15 units of regular insulin about 15 minutes before each meal. I don't remember how many calories I was allowed, but I do remember being constantly hungry and "thin as a rail." I was 13 years old and beginning to grow rapidly, yet no changes were made to my diet to provide nutrition for my rapid growth. I was told that I should not exercise vigorously. My mother was told that I should be permanently excused from "gym classes." As we now know, this was unnecessary, and in fact, bad advice.

Dr. Eaddy says: In 1952, when I was diagnosed, diet colas were hard to find and usually cost more than $1.00 a bottle—which was expensive! Soon after being diagnosed, I remember being with a group of teen-age friends at a neighborhood drug store fountain. Everyone but me was ordering banana splits, ice cream sodas, and other delicious high-calorie treats. I can still remember how they made fun of me because I ordered a milk float. My doctor had told me this would be an acceptable treat. It was, but that didn't help my feelings.

The rigid diet prescribed years ago caused many problems. It was difficult for most people to weigh or measure portions of foods for every meal. How do you do that when you eat in the school or company cafeteria or go out to a restaurant? Who knew how many calories were in servings of casseroles or pizzas purchased in supermarkets, restaurants, or baked at home? In addition, we longed to eat what other people ate. We didn't like being "special."

Nowadays, we can eat what everyone else eats. A healthy diet is a healthy diet for everyone. We know a great deal more about the nutrients in foods—especially carbohydrate, protein, and fat—and how they affect blood glucose levels. We have books and food labels that give us all the nutrition information for a serving of food. We can count carbohydrates in our meals to control our blood sugar. Occasionally we get out the food scale or the measuring cup to be sure of our serving sizes. We have a wealth of nutrition information that makes meal planning much simpler—and tastier—for people with diabetes.

Eating the same foods

Before we had as much help from the experts as we do today, we depended a lot on consistency to keep our caloric intake within bounds. Dr. Lincoln remembers: I usually ate three vegetables, a Jello salad with a tablespoon of French dressing, and one scoop of sherbet every noon at the company cafeteria where I worked. It may not have been the diet prescribed, but at least it was consistent. I could adjust my insulin dose to it. This was before home blood glucose monitoring was available, but I checked my urine glucose occasionally to see how I was doing. It wasn't very exact but I did reasonably well. Since the vegetables sometimes had sauces or pasta, the calorie content of my noon meal was not always the same. As a precaution, I took a little extra insulin to cover it and then had a snack later in the afternoon when my blood glucose might be getting too low.

Needless to say, I had a good many episodes of mild hypoglycemia that I controlled by eating candy or going to the department refrigerator for something to drink. The evening meal was the most difficult because I craved variety. Here again, I took a little extra insulin and then checked my urine glucose at bedtime. I had more than my share of severe episodes of hypoglycemia at night in spite of eating a snack before I went to bed. Fortunately, my wife was always able to rescue me.

New Insulin Brings New Benefits and New Challenges

In the 1950s, it became popular to use slow-acting insulin. We could get by with only one injection a day. There was better control of blood glucose toward morning because the regular insulin previously taken before supper only lasted about 6–8 hours. The problem was that the very slowness of the intermediate-acting insulin created a potential hazard. Once we took the injection in the morning, a relatively slow but continuous insulin action would take place throughout the day and into the night. Blood glucose would slowly fall too low, causing hypoglycemia. In those days, we adjusted to this problem by modifications in our diet. When we expected blood glucose to be lowest, such as in the late afternoon, we would eat an afternoon snack to prevent hypoglycemia.

Nowadays, in the intensive management of diabetes, it is common to take rapid-acting insulin before each meal and then take long-acting insulin in the morning before breakfast or at bedtime. This type of diabetes management allows you much more flexibility and provides much better control of your blood glucose. Here again, meal planning plays a crucial role. You know when to expect your blood glucose to be lowest and can eat a small snack if you are beginning to feel like you're going too low. Of course, you might be able to check your blood glucose to get more specific information so you can decide whether to have a snack. You can count the grams of carbohydrate (carb) in the meal before you go low and take less insulin or eat more carb to prevent low blood sugar.

Choices, we've got choices

To manage your own diabetes, you need to develop some skill in selecting the foods you will eat. Food raises blood glucose. Exercise and medication lower it. We use food to stay healthy, get energy, and prevent and treat low blood sugar. Learning about the nutrients in foods and how to choose a healthy meal is important, and you need help with developing a meal plan that fits your food likes and dislikes, your schedule, your family, and your health goals. You should meet with a registered dietitian (RD) to create your meal plan and learn about serving sizes and the nutrients in foods. This is important when you are diagnosed, but it is also important when things change: you go from one life stage to another, start exercising more, go off to college or retire, get pregnant, or have problems with low blood sugars that you can't explain. Your meal plan is a valuable tool, so be sure you use it well.

Health care team?

Your family physician may refer you to a RD for help with your meal planning. The RD may also be a certified diabetes educator (CDE), which means that she has special training in diabetes management and can help you with yours. Nurses (RN, BSN) can also be CDEs and are often your contact at the doctor's office for help with diabetes management training and questions. Other health care professionals, such as doctors (MD, DO), psychologists (PhD), and counselors (MSW, LCSW) can become certified diabetes educators, too.

To get the best diabetes care, you are fortunate if you have one or all of these professionals on your "health care team." Most diabetes education centers at large hospitals have diabetes care teams of professionals. If you don't have a center near you, you may have to build your own team. You can find qualified professionals at your local hospital, health department, or medical clinic. You can call the ADA to get their list of Recognized Providers who follow the ADA Standards of Care for treating people with diabetes. You can ask other people with diabetes who is on their team.

You are the most important member of your health care team. You are the expert on you, and the professionals are your advisors in managing your own diabetes. To become expert on yourself, you need to be willing to keep records of your meals, blood glucose levels, and insulin doses. You take these records to your health care advisors to figure out the best way to take care of your diabetes, given your lifestyle, schedule, and needs. Without your records, no decisions can be made. As you learn about yourself and gain experience with diabetes, you will learn to adjust your insulin dose based on your food intake, insulin, and blood glucose levels. You can be flexible enough to do things on the spur of the moment, to put off meals, or to eat larger than usual meals and still keep your blood glucose levels near normal. Or if you don't want to try intensive management (tight control), your health will still benefit from what you learn about yourself and your diabetes. Some people don't try for tight control for various reasons, such as weight gain, increased episodes of severe hypoglycemia, and the problem of getting the necessary professional advice and training. These problems can be controlled.

What to Do With a Meal Plan

Fortunately, most people eat the same foods from week to week—the menus don't vary much, so these are the foods that will probably go into your meal plan. A meal plan helps you get breakfast, lunch, and dinner meals of approximately the same size each day. This helps bring a pattern to your daily blood glucose levels. From that point, you can begin to substitute other foods and use snacks to help you bring variety to your meal plan without risking low blood sugar. You're also learning how much medication and how much exercise keep your blood glucose levels where you want them.

Some people, however, find this intensive management responsibility overwhelming. They don't know enough about food values. They don't know how to substitute other foods when something is not available. If they make a mistake and overeat and discover that their blood glucose is high, they don't know how much extra rapid-acting insulin to take. Don't despair. Be patient with yourself and do the best you can (Table 7-1). With these experiences—frustrating as some of them may be—you are learning how to manage your own diabetes. And that's important. Get the help of your health care providers. Read about meal planning. Get some healthy cookbooks. Enjoy choosing what you will eat.

The power to overeat

When you begin to assume responsibility for adjusting your own insulin, you will be tempted to supplement your insulin

---

TABLE 7-1

Hints for Healthy Eating

- Grocery shop when you are not hungry, and use a shopping list.
- Learn to read and understand food labels.
- Avoid the temptations of the deli.
- Eat high-quality snacks such as fresh fruit or vegetables. Don't depend on candy, cookies, or snacks that are high in fat, salt, and calories.
- Don't bring home the high-fat, high-salt, high-calorie snacks.
- Eat only in the kitchen or dining room, not in front of the TV or in bed. Try to eat at scheduled meals and snack times.

dose to meet your desire for high-calorie foods. When you take extra insulin, your blood glucose will more frequently fall to low levels. One of the most common early symptoms of mild hypoglycemia is hunger. As you chase your low blood glucose by eating more sweet foods, you are going to gain weight. If you don't want to gain weight, don't take supplementary insulin any more often than necessary—that is to say, don't overindulge in big meals and lots of dessert so that you need the extra insulin.

If you use tight control, you must always be prepared for low blood sugar. Carry insulin, a glucose meter, and foods to treat lows with you at all times.

Teenagers and food and insulin

Some young people on intensive management run into a vicious cycle, often called "brittle" diabetes. Adolescents' blood glucose levels tend to go up and down faster than adults. It is part of rapid growth and development. In girls, it can be related to the menstrual cycle. Teens with brittle diabetes often take too little insulin at a meal, so they can have flexibility in their eating. But then, they wind up with high blood glucose. Then they take extra insulin to counteract the high and wind up later with another low blood glucose. Around and around they go, gaining weight in the process.

Some teens use their insulin to lose weight. They take too little for a meal so they'll have high blood glucose to lose the glucose and calories in their urine. This is a very dangerous practice. These are the teens we see too often in the hospital emergency room in ketoacidosis and impending coma. These young people risk their lives now and increase their risk of developing complications early in their lives.

Type 2 and meal plan concerns

People with type 2 are not insulin dependent, but about 40% of you will progress to using insulin to control your blood glucose better. Some people with type 2 can control blood glucose with meal planning and exercise alone. Some people require one or more diabetes pills to lower blood sugar. All people with type 2 diabetes must follow a meal plan, get exercise, and may need to take insulin for the best control. A lot of people delay going on insulin and spend more years with high blood sugar than they need to. Large research studies have shown that good control of blood sugar is as important in preventing complications for people with type 2 as it is for people with type 1 diabetes. If you need insulin, don't delay. You'll feel better soon.

Hypoglycemia is a concern if you are on any medicine that lowers blood glucose. Among the diabetes pills, those that can cause hypoglycemia are the sulfonylureas, repaglinide, nateglinide, and the combination of glyburide and metformin. Because hypoglycemia is less frequent in type 2 patients, the tendency for both patients and doctors is to be relaxed. This can be dangerous. Keeping track of blood glucose levels is still important. HbA1c tests should be done once or twice a year. You may not need to check your blood glucose at home as often as people using insulin do, but you should check whenever you have eaten a larger than normal meal or exercised a lot. You need to know where your blood sugar level is and what to do about it to raise or lower it.

Food tips

You will learn from both your successes and your mistakes. The following food tips may help:

1. Remember that some foods take much longer to digest and be absorbed and, therefore, to increase your blood glucose. It is possible to have a mild hypoglycemic episode even though you have already eaten some meat or fatty food. If you feel low when you sit down at the table, eat something that is quickly absorbed. Have some soda containing sugar, some fruit juice, bread, potatoes, or rice.

2. The best way to gain control of your blood glucose is to be consistent in your eating habits.

3. Remember that exercise will often lower your blood glucose quickly. You should carry some carbohydrate food with you. If you have mildly high glucose, go for a vigorous walk before you eat. If your blood glucose monitor reads over 300, get your glucose under control before you exercise. You will probably need to take a small amount of rapid-acting insulin.

4. Don't take rapid-acting or short-acting insulin and then go for a vigorous walk, because your blood glucose can fall remarkably fast.

5. Be prepared for any possible mishap. Have some type of candy or sugar in one pocket and a bottle of rapid-acting or regular insulin and a syringe or insulin pen in the other pocket before you leave home each day.

   Yes, insulin should be refrigerated, but it is stable at room temperature for one month after the bottle is opened. If it is carried around in warm weather and loses strength, the loss is small. You never know when you will need either food or insulin: traffic jams, storms, working overtime, car accident, subway delay, etc. Have reserve supplies of candy or glucose in your car and workplace.

6. Eat slowly. Give your food a chance to be digested, absorbed, and start to raise your blood sugar so you can feel full before you overeat.

7. Watch low-fat and low-sugar foods. They are not free foods. The manufacturers have to use more carbohydrate to make low-fat foods taste good, and that carbohydrate will raise your blood sugar. This applies to low-fat salad dressings as well as to cookies. Check the calorie and carb count of low-sugar foods, too. You don't want to be surprised.

8. Artificial sweeteners are clearly useful. There is no need to be concerned about safety in using them. The Food and Drug Administration (FDA) has determined safe amounts that can be added to foods. Remember never to try to treat hypoglycemia with a diet drink—it won't work.

8

What Exercise Does for Blood Sugar

Physical activity has a profound effect on your blood glucose level. Activities such as mowing the lawn, working in the garden, or taking a brisk walk have caused many low blood sugar levels in people who did not know better. You might think, then, that exercise should be avoided. Nothing could be further from the truth! Exercise is one of the most important parts of treatment for every one of us. You can easily avoid the hazards of hypoglycemia once you understand what is happening when you exercise.

The Benefits of Exercise

Exercise is unique in its favorable effects on diabetes—and many people use it with a meal plan to manage their diabetes. The benefits of exercise include preventing heart disease, improving circulation, maintaining strength in bones and joints, and reducing emotional tension. You can use exercise to lower blood glucose and to work off extra calories. You can use it with meal planning to lose weight and keep it off.

Keeping your heart healthy. People with diabetes are likely to have problems with circulation, heart disease, and high blood pressure (hypertension). You can use exercise to prevent these problems from developing. Regular exercise causes a decrease in bad cholesterol (low-density lipoproteins [LDL]). These are the fats that may be deposited in the lining of your arteries and gradually obstruct them. If the blockage becomes severe enough, it may cause heart attacks or reduced blood supply to your feet, brain, or heart.

Vigorous exercise raises high-density lipoproteins (HDL), the good cholesterol, which helps protect arteries against future deposits of fat. These benefits are achieved when you exercise several days a week for 30 minutes or more each day.

Regular exercise has a favorable effect on high blood pressure and reduces the resting pulse rate. It increases the work capacity of the heart muscle. People who get regular physical exercise usually tolerate a heart attack much better than people who have led a sedentary lifestyle. Regular exercise helps protect the heart from stresses that might precipitate a chaotic rhythm disturbance, the most common cardiac cause of sudden death.

Regular exercise has a favorable effect on the development of collateral circulation around a developing blockage in an artery. The vigorous use of muscle groups during exercise requires a great increase in the flow of blood to these muscles to supply nourishment and oxygen. When this happens, small arteries dilate to allow more blood to flow through them. This dilation with exercise (and constriction with rest) tends to keep arteries open better and allows new collateral branches to develop around an artery that is becoming blocked.

Everyone has heard of middle-aged men having fatal heart attacks while they are exercising. The popular conclusion is that had they not been exercising, they might still be alive. An explanation that is more reasonable is that the previous exercise may have provided years of protection. Without exercise, the victim might have had a heart attack years earlier.

Muscles and joints. Exercise provides strength to muscles and helps maintain flexibility in joints. Use keeps them from getting rusty. People who get regular exercise tend to have less arthritis. Degenerative arthritis that develops especially in the hips, knees, and ankles is largely a metabolic and genetic disease. Athletic injuries to joints may predispose you to develop degenerative arthritis, but reasonable exercise does not cause arthritis. Exercise may aggravate a specific arthritic joint and may have to be restricted in some cases. Inflamed or swollen joints should be exercised very carefully and only under medical supervision.

Emotions and muscles. Exercise has many psychological benefits and is particularly valuable for people under emotional stress. It will give you a sense of well-being and enhanced self-esteem. Regular aerobic exercise helps many people ward off feelings of depression and lightens their mood. Stress and depression can play havoc with your blood glucose, usually making it too high. Besides aerobic exercise, other types of exercise, such as yoga or tai chi, help you stretch and relax and help lower blood glucose levels, too.

What Exercise Does

Understanding a few facts about how the body works will help you avoid hypoglycemia during exercise. During exercise, our muscles propel us and enable us to lift objects. When you are sitting quietly, your muscles get only about 10% of their energy from burning glucose. At rest, most of the energy is provided by burning fatty acids derived from fat. When you start to walk, muscles quickly require much more fuel. This fuel is provided by burning glucose. As you walk fairly briskly, there is a rapid increase in blood delivered to your muscles to provide more oxygen to burn the glucose.

In people who don't have diabetes, as glucose is burned in muscles, it is replaced by glucose released from the liver. The pancreas slows down the release of insulin. A beautiful control mechanism keeps a constant level of glucose circulating in the blood to supply the working muscles and the brain. This wonderful system enables conditioned athletes to run 25 miles and never experience any significant hypoglycemia.

If you have injected insulin, however, there is no way to turn it off when you are exercising. After jogging for a mile or two, your blood glucose comes down because exercise is burning it while using very little insulin. Soon you have an excess of insulin, and your blood glucose begins to fall too low. The obvious answer is to take less insulin or to eat more carbohydrate at the meal before you exercise. However, with the different action times of insulin and the fact that few people exercise exactly the same amount at the same time each day, it is difficult to predict the effect exercise will have on your blood sugar. Making an adjustment to your insulin is tricky, and you do need some insulin while you're exercising, so most people choose to prevent low blood sugar by carrying food or juice to snack on when they start to go too low.

An exercised muscle

Remember that exercise can make the insulin you inject go into action more quickly if you are exercising the body part where you injected. For example, if you are a runner, you should not inject into your thighs or calves. Inject your insulin into your abdomen. If you exercise after eating and you have taken insulin 15–30 minutes before the meal, there usually has been time for enough of your food to be digested and absorbed so your blood glucose has risen to an adequate level. Some of you may be shocked by this advice to exercise after eating. Walking or jogging after eating is safe and comfortable. Your blood glucose is rising as the food is being digested.

Exercise before a meal, especially the evening meal, can be especially hazardous if you are taking intermediate-acting insulin, such as NPH or lente, before breakfast. This early evening time is when the insulin is reaching its peak. Even though your blood glucose was normal before starting exercise, it can fall rapidly during the exercise.

It is generally accepted that you should not exercise when your blood glucose is over 300 mg/dl. On the other hand, if you are in pretty good control but have high blood glucose on a single test, you can exercise as an easy way of getting your glucose down to a more normal level. We often hear it described as "running down" a high glucose late in the afternoon before the evening meal. Perhaps because of eating something as a safety precaution before driving home, you will find your blood glucose to be over 200 mg/dl when you get home. If you run or walk for 45 minutes, your glucose level may decline to near normal by dinnertime.

If your blood glucose is over 250 mg/dl, check your urine for ketones. If ketones are present, don't exercise until you can get them down to only trace amounts. Talk with your health care providers about the best way to handle this situation.

What You Do

By checking your blood glucose level each time before and after you exercise, you can learn how much your glucose will come down during a planned exercise. You soon learn how much extra food is necessary to cover a specific amount of exercise. It is much more difficult when you plan to play a strenuous game such as tennis or basketball. The amount of energy you expend depends on how hard and how long you play, and on how hot or cold it is. Of course, the same could be said of going outdoors to mow the lawn or shovel snow off the driveway.

Prevention tips

Always keep a supply of candy or sweet beverages with you so you can raise your blood sugar if it starts falling too low. Dr. Lincoln and his wife were walking on a vacation out in the country. After about 3 miles, Dr. Lincoln began to get weak and feel that he was going low. He couldn't walk well enough to get back to the house, so his wife sat him down by the side of the road and ran back the remaining mile to the house. Fortunately, he obeyed and stayed there until she drove back with orange juice for him. He recovered in a few minutes, but they were both scared and realized how foolish they had been to walk so far without having a snack or money to buy one, if one had been available. He says, "From that day on, I never leave home without carrying candy in a small plastic bag in one of my pockets."

You may have been walking or running for years with no problems, but that doesn't mean you won't go low tomorrow. Usually hypoglycemia shows up early or later during exercise depending on the vigor of the exercise and where your glucose was when you started. The earliest symptoms are unusual tiredness, muscle fatigue, and declining skill. Learn from the next two stories and watch for the signs in yourself.

A patient told us: One time when I was in my early 40s, I developed the following problem. I tried to swim a mile each evening with my goal of reaching 50 miles during the summer. I would swim 16 laps using a relatively slow freestyle stroke. Even though I always had eaten my evening meal before I went swimming, on several occasions I found myself struggling and using a wildly unusual stroke. I had to stop even though I was not aware that I was hypoglycemic. I thought my mind was clear, and I felt good. I had something to eat because I became sure that I must be slightly hypoglycemic. Although my glucose must have returned to normal, I found that it took so long to restore my skill that I had to give up and go home.

Muscle efforts that require a high level of skill and coordination are the very first to be impaired by low blood glucose and take the longest to return. This decline in skill can often be the first sign of a falling blood glucose. Here's another example.

A retired executive told us that he could tell when his glucose was getting low because his golf score would climb rapidly. Although he usually felt normal, his golf partners said he became very talkative and lost his concentration when putting or making a drive. He made several of his golfing partners unhappy because they would recognize that he was getting low blood glucose, and it was affecting his score, but he often resisted doing anything about it.

This man could do himself (and his golf buddies) a big favor if he accepted a worsening score as a sign of low blood sugar and ate several glucose tablets that he carries with him. There's no place to get something to eat on the back side of a golf course.

Hours later

The glucose-lowering effect of exercise continues to act for many hours after you have finished exercising, even into the next day. This is a benefit of exercise, but be aware that severe hypoglycemia may occur during the night 12 hours after exercise. Such episodes are more likely in young people and in people on vacation, when exercise is often unplanned and vigorous and eating is not normal. Bedtime blood glucose checks can alert you to eat a larger than usual snack before you go to bed to avoid going too low.

Diabetes pills and exercise

If you are taking any diabetes pills, you should be alert for low blood sugar during exercise. It can happen. It is most likely to happen to people who take sulfonylureas, repaglinide, or nateglinide. You get the same benefits from exercise and need to take the same precautions. In fact, all people with diabetes should be delighted in and prepared for the blood glucose–lowering effects of the healthy activities they pursue.

Prevention!

There is now impressive evidence that regular exercise helps prevent type 2 diabetes in both men and women. This protection may be related to the consistently lower blood glucose levels because of exercise! Patients with type 2 who exercise have lower HbA1c levels, and this means better glucose control. Exercise is the magic key when it comes to keeping diabetes under control.

9

Handling Lows at School

Most cases of type 1 diabetes develop in children between the ages of 9 and 14, during the school years. Having hypoglycemia in school is a major worry for both parents and children. Although everyone will try hard to prevent this from happening, it is reasonable to expect that all children with diabetes will eventually have several reactions while at school.

Elementary School Kids

Elementary school children are pretty responsible about snacking when they need to and taking care of their diabetes. Send them to school every day with a cooler or backpack full of the things they need: insulin, syringe or pen, glucose meter, strips, foods for snacks, and foods to treat low blood sugar. Give a sheet to the teacher listing the symptoms of low blood sugar and what to do for your child if they happen. Include a sheet with your emergency phone numbers on it, too.

Some school administrators may object to assuming any responsibility for helping to manage students with diabetes.

However, several federal laws protect school children with diabetes. They include Section 504 of the Rehabilitation Act of 1973, the Individuals with Disabilities Act of 1991, and the Americans with Disabilities Act of 1992. Under these laws, diabetes has been determined to be a disability and schools cannot discriminate against children with this disease. The responsibilities of each player in this problem have been defined in an ADA Position Statement (Care of Children with Diabetes in the School and Day Care Setting). To get a copy, call 1-800-DIABETES. You, your physician, and the school authorities should read it before school starts.

Before school each year, you need to set up a meeting with your child's physician, teacher, and the principal to develop an individualized diabetes care plan. This plan should include the specific needs of your child and define who is expected to do what to help prevent and treat episodes of hypoglycemia. You can get an example plan form from ADA. With the plan done, you need to meet with and explain to the teachers, principal, school nurse, and any other staff who will interact with your child the basics about diabetes and what they can do to help your child if he goes too low. You might also provide the teacher with a stash of foods for your child, should she need them. Most school nurses are not on duty all day every day, so the teacher is your most important link. Warn the staff of your child's symptoms of low blood sugar and that he may be aggressive in resisting help. A hypoglycemic episode can be an emotional event; if you prepare them, it is likely to turn out better for all concerned.

You might also take that opportunity to tell them two things about food. First, your child will need to eat snacks during the day, every day, to prevent low blood sugar, and they should make sure that the child can do this and feels free to do it. It will take some explaining for your child's classmates to understand that he needs to eat at certain times or he will get sick—and that he's not getting a treat that they aren't getting. Then tell them that your child can eat birthday cake, so please not to single her out in front of the class as having to eat only certain foods. Kids with diabetes can eat everything that other kids eat.

By law, children with diabetes must be accepted into the classroom and provisions made for their special needs, such as letting them eat those snacks at 10 and 2. You may have difficulty, however, finding a teacher who is willing to help your child check her blood glucose. Many people are reluctant to do it, so it's wise not to press the issue. A poorly done test is no help anyway. If your child is capable of checking his own glucose, set up with the teacher and principal where and when he can do this.

Your child must feel comfortable approaching the teacher about feeling low or eating an unscheduled snack if she feels that she is going low. The teacher should understand the need not to delay getting juice or glucose tablets into your child. Reassure the teacher and the other staff that your child's condition will improve in about 10 minutes. Ask them not to panic and run to call home or an ambulance and delay taking care of the child. If the child does not improve in 10 or 15 minutes, the teacher should give her more juice or regular soda. It isn't reasonable to expect a teacher to be able to give a glucagon injection.

It helps if you also teach your child's friends about diabetes and what to do when he goes too low. Friends can speak up for your child when she can't. A friend should always accompany your child if he is going to the nurse or to the office with low blood sugar—otherwise your child might not be able to get there.

Timing is everything

Teachers are frequently unaware of the importance of timing of meals and snacks. They don't appreciate what suddenly changing the time of a meal or snack can do to a child with diabetes. They don't appreciate how class trips during the day, for example, a trip to an art museum or the zoo, can upset eating schedules and increase the danger of hypoglycemia. You can help prepare your child by talking in advance about necessary changes in food or insulin. Teachers are also frequently unaware that physical exercise (chapter 8) during classes or games during lunchtime can have a big effect on a student's blood glucose level. Your child needs regular exercise to be healthy, but teachers should be alert for symptoms of low blood sugar during and for several hours after.

Doing Well on Tests

If your child is even mildly hypoglycemic, she may not do well on achievement or intelligence tests. The stress of taking an exam can cause blood glucose to drop, and your child needs to be aware of this. A snack before or during the test might be a good idea. If your child tells the teacher that she is having trouble with low blood glucose right away, she may be able to snack and then take the test, or to take it later when she is feeling clearheaded.

It is also important to consider the potential effects of high blood glucose on students. High blood glucose slows down thinking processes and mathematical ability. The student seems lethargic and slow. If your child's performance at school is declining, then you and your child's teachers need to discuss the effects that low and high blood glucose may be having on him.

Adolescents

You may be surprised to learn that school nurses report many more difficulties for adolescents dealing with their diabetes, or not dealing with it. Most adolescents do not want to stand out as different from their friends. They will go to great lengths to hide the fact that they have diabetes and have to eat at certain times, check their blood glucose, and take their insulin. It is a time of rebellion and of acting out, so diabetes care often suffers as a result. Many teenagers choose to let their blood glucose run high to avoid having to deal with hypoglycemia in front of other students. The fear of future complications is not as strong as the fear of having an embarrassing episode in front of classmates or teammates at school.

Of course, you want to respect your child's wishes, but secrecy is not the best policy when her health is at risk. Her teachers and at least one close friend should know the symptoms of low blood glucose and what to do to treat it. The teachers need to know that it is okay for your child to be eating in class, so they won't draw attention to what he is doing. If your child needs to eat to avoid going too low, then get support for him to take care of his diabetes before he needs it.

10

Teenagers and the Blood Sugar Blues

Type 1 diabetes most frequently appears during adolescence, a time when a child has to make many adjustments to deal with puberty and the responsibilities that come with growing up. Diabetes further complicates things. You and your child will decide how and when to tell others about his diabetes, but you must know that your decision will have an effect on how well he handles diabetes during these years. Adolescents feel alone and awkward much of the time, even when they don't have diabetes. If you can make diabetes as much a part of the natural schedule and routine of the household as possible, it will help your child.

We discussed handling diabetes at school in chapter 9. We know many teenagers who are comfortable enough to inject insulin in class or the lunchroom if they need to. Rebecca Shacklett is a good example. She has had diabetes for 8 years, since she was 8 years old. She says, "When I'm giving myself a shot, people who don't know me always ask, 'Doesn't that hurt?' But the most common question is 'Why do you get to eat whenever you want?' I answer, 'Because I have diabetes.'"

This paragraph and the next reflect Rebecca's viewpoint of when hypoglycemia is a problem for adolescents. Diabetes is not as difficult for your child in the classroom as it is out on the athletic field and on trips. Playing sports burns glucose rapidly, so your child and your child's coaches—and the other team members—need to know the symptoms of low blood sugar and how to treat it. Your child must always carry snack foods and glucose tablets to practices and to games and use them. The other players may give her trouble about getting to come out of the game to eat—as Rebecca's friends do—but she can explain that it is to protect her against going too low. Hopefully, they'll soon join in helping her avoid hypoglycemia. Diabetes will not interfere with her ability to be a good athlete. In fact, sports help adolescents through the passage to adulthood, by easing stress and building self-confidence. Your child should play.

When you're traveling, it's difficult to exercise while you're sitting in a car or on a plane. Most people don't have problems with low blood sugar on a trip—it's more common to have high blood glucose. So, your child may want to take a little bit of extra insulin. Talk with your health care provider about how best to do this. And of course, your child should carry snack foods, and maybe a complete meal, with him. You never know when there will be a delay, or he will go low and need to eat.

What you know

It will help you and your adolescent to know about the things that can affect his blood sugar levels. Anything that can help take the mystery out of blood sugar patterns will keep the frustration level down.

Sexual Development

Sex hormones have major effects on blood glucose levels. Sex hormones are on the rise during puberty. A girl's first menstrual period represents the external sign of profound changes that are taking place in her body. A boy doesn't have a single sexual event, other than possibly his first ejaculation, that signals his arrival at puberty. Nevertheless, by this time the secretion of sex hormones from the ovaries in the girl and the testicles in the boy have already had huge effects on growth and development.

Boys and girls who develop diabetes before puberty are often disappointed and frustrated because their puberty and growth are delayed. The years of puberty (11–14) are the most common time that type 1 diabetes appears. Since puberty already requires some major psychological and physical adjustments, it is particularly difficult to superimpose the new adjustment problems of diabetes on top of all these other concerns.

The slowness to grow and sexually mature in adolescent boys and girls is clearly related to poor control of the diabetes. We used to think that this difficulty in controlling diabetes was due to the emotional turmoil that frequently accompanies puberty. In recent years, several studies have shown that normal growth and development in adolescents who don't have diabetes also cause disturbances in glucose metabolism. For example, during puberty in every adolescent, insulin resistance develops. The pancreas has to produce more insulin to metabolize normal amounts of food. This insulin resistance automatically disappears after a few years. In the diabetic adolescent, insulin resistance may be related to the large amounts of growth hormone that are released during puberty.

Regardless of the cause, puberty is a time when tight control of blood glucose levels is extremely difficult. More insulin has to be injected, and blood glucose levels seem to bounce around from high to low. Young women with diabetes frequently have difficulty controlling their glucose during menstrual periods, especially 1–3 days before the beginning of the period and then during the first 3–5 days of the period.

Adolescents with diabetes who struggle to maintain tight control of their diabetes often experience many episodes of hypoglycemia. Both parents and adolescents get discouraged and relax their efforts at control, hoping that treatment will be easier after a few years. It eventually is easier, but 6–8 years of poor control can greatly increase the likelihood of the early onset of complications.

Those lucky adolescents who are encouraged to assume most of the responsibility for the management of their diabetes and are helped to learn from their mistakes often do remarkably well. Those who are only told what to do can easily blame their parents or doctors for their failures. Reassure your adolescent that learning how to control diabetes is no more difficult than learning to become an expert swimmer or basketball player. In all three, you learn basic skills from an expert, spend thousands of hours in practice, learn from mistakes, and have a great desire to win.

Gaining Independence

Before puberty, children are reasonably comfortable depending on their parents for guidance and protection. As puberty progresses, questioning parental authority becomes increasingly common. This questioning includes the authority to manage their disease.

Parents are frequently afraid to delegate control of meal planning, insulin, and physical activities to their maturing child. The effect on the child is summed up in this complaint from a 15-year-old boy. "How can I get my parents to let me have more responsibilities? I'm diabetic, and they won't even let me go to my grandparents' house for lunch. Usually on weekends I have to stay inside from 9:45 p.m. till 7 a.m. when I get up." Isn't it better to give him the tools he needs and to let him practice using them before he goes off to college or gets a job and moves away from home?

In many respects, young people with diabetes must learn to become their own physicians, their own laboratory technicians, and their own nurses. Helping adolescents develop enough skill to manage their own diabetes is difficult for parents because they frequently are insecure about their own capabilities. But it's a time for you all to learn. We've learned that high rather than low blood glucose levels are what happens when parents let go of the diabetes management chores too quickly. The handoff process should be slow and steady and timed to your child's demonstrated successes. Even if your child does it perfectly, there will still be occasional episodes of poor control. All kids have to be given the opportunity to learn from their own experiences.

Parents often fail to remember their own adolescence. Many young people break forcefully from their parent's control with fierce arguments and pathological behavior. If there's a family fight, expect some future episodes of severe hypoglycemia or hyperglycemia.

To hide it or not to hide it?

Parents seldom get a chance to hear their adolescents ventilate about what bothers them. Although it was 50 years ago, Dr. Lincoln remembers vividly his concerns.

I wanted desperately to be one of the gang. (Gangs had different activities when I was growing up.) Physically, I had no deformities, and I could keep my diabetes a secret. I found that most difficult when I had to eat with my friends. I said. "I'm not hungry," when sugary snacks and Cokes were being passed around. At mealtimes, I tried to approximate my usual meal from what I was offered. I never told my friends about taking insulin. I was extremely careful to avoid hypoglycemia. I began early to take a little extra regular insulin when I went with my friends to the popular diner after a high school basketball game.

Nothing was more upsetting to me than to have a parent of a friend of mine remind my friends that "Tommy can't eat that because he is a diabetic." The idea that I was "different" hurt me more than anything else. Early in my adolescence, I became determined that I was going to control my diabetes without my friends ever knowing what I was doing. I continued this "silence" all the way through medical school, telling only a few essential people. This determination to be independent forced me to study closely the effect of what I ate, how much more or less insulin I could take under special circumstances, and what vigorous exercise would do to cause me to have hypoglycemia attacks. Back then, I only had urine sugar tests, which I soon learned were not very reliable. I used the frequency of mild hypoglycemia as the measure of when I was probably under reasonable control. When I had to urinate frequently, I knew my blood sugar must be high. I did occasionally test my urine for sugar but when the test was bright red, I had no idea just how high my blood glucose level was. I just knew it must be real high!

I learned very quickly that no so-called expert would be of great help. I could get valuable general advice but daily decisions were my parent's and my responsibility. I had to try everything and sometimes fail in order to learn. I made many mistakes but my survival and good health to age 76 is evidence of my success.

Straight Talk to Teens

Now with blood glucose testing so easy, it might be even easier to hide your diabetes from everyone except your closest friends and a few others who have to know. You could test your blood glucose in a rest room and decide how much you needed to eat or whether you needed to adjust your dosage of regular insulin. But being too secretive with your diabetes can be hazardous, and we don't recommend you do that. Better to develop the self-confidence to be casual and open with your friends about your invisible handicap.

You have to fight the same battles that all adolescents do to succeed in "growing up." Under these challenges, some kids get pessimistic and withdraw. But, many more kids with diabetes mature emotionally earlier than their friends.

Young people have to grow up the best way that they can. Those who have good family support will probably do well. Those who have broken and chaotic family lives will have more challenges, but many do remarkably well. Probably the most practical suggestion is to test your blood glucose frequently by yourself. Don't depend on your parents to push you or do it for you. Make the decision that you are going to be the boss of your disease. You are going to learn how to figure out your glucose patterns, so you can go anywhere with your friends, eat when they eat, play when they play, and enjoy a full rich life.

11

Sex, Pregnancy, and Hypoglycemia

Diabetes can have an effect on your sexual health, both in your ability to physically enjoy it and to feel like enjoying it. Good glucose control prevents the nerve and circulation damage that can interfere with a man's ability to have an erection and a woman's ability to have an orgasm. And it can improve your health and emotional state so you are in the right frame of mind to enjoy sex. In healthy men and women, sexual orgasm is a complicated neurological (nerves and brain), psychological (emotions and thoughts), and physiological (physical) function. It is easily impaired by alcohol, drugs, poor circulation, diabetes, and other chronic diseases, especially neurological disorders.

The key to the prevention of impaired sexual performance in both men and women is tight control of blood glucose. People who maintain an HbA1c below 7% (chapter 4) most of the time during the many years of their disease will have much less difficulty with their sex lives.

Since sexual functioning depends on healthy thoughts, nerves, and blood vessels, all three systems must be working well to accomplish pleasurable sexual activity. In either males or females, fatigue, feeling sick, depression, and severe anxiety can also interfere with sexual desire and performance. You need to evaluate your own mental state when sexual performance or desire fails. If you are worried that you will have low blood sugar while you are having sex, you are not likely to enjoy it or to participate well. And your partner, with whom you may not have shared your fears, will feel puzzled or rejected—causing problems for the next time. Of course, having hypoglycemia during sex can be embarrassing and frustrating and impact your sex life, too.

Sexual activity is like any physical exercise. You can go too low during or after. You may check your blood glucose before sex, especially if you think you might be going low. In any case, you can eat a small snack before and have some food available in case you need it during or right after. If your blood glucose does go low during sex, you are likely to lose sensation and lubrication. The magic of the moment is lost and is difficult to recapture at the moment. It is probably best to try again later. See Table 11-1 for ways to prepare for a good sexual relationship.

Like other people, diabetic men and women are often extremely reluctant to discuss sexual performance with their physicians. Likewise, many physicians are so uncomfortable with the subject that they never ask their patients about it. There is much that can be done. If you are having difficulty, please ask your physician to refer you to an expert for help.

Pregnancy

If you want to become pregnant, it is important for your health and for the health of your newborn child to start getting good control of your diabetes right away—before you are pregnant. As we've said before, when you are striving for tight

TABLE 11-1

Ways to Create a Good Sexual Relationship

1. Maintain good glucose control.

2. Exercise regularly.

3. When erection or sensation problems appear to be developing, discuss your concerns with the doctor who helps you with your diabetes.

4. Check blood glucose before going to bed. Have a small snack if it is 110–125 mg/dl or less.

5. Infections of bladder, kidneys, or genitals should be treated promptly and correctly.

6. Partners should periodically discuss the love-sexual relationship at a time when resentment, anger, and anxiety are under control. Seek professional help for problems that can't be easily resolved.

control of your blood glucose, you are going to have more episodes of low blood sugar, so be ready for them.

The risk of hypoglycemia is greatest during the first half of pregnancy. Women often have decreased awareness of their early symptoms of hypoglycemia, which leads, of course, to the episodes being more severe when they occur. Morning sickness and other digestive disturbances make control more difficult. It appears that you have an increased sensitivity to the effects of insulin, and the sensitivity may vary at different times during the pregnancy.

Glucagon (made by the body) and other counter-regulatory hormones that normally help the body react to low blood glucose are not produced as much during pregnancy. Glucagon production declines during the first 5–10 years of type 1 diabetes anyway, so if you've had diabetes this length of time and you are pregnant, your glucagon response may be at a very low level (chapter 5).

Pregnant women need to check their blood glucose up to 8 or 10 times a day. The good outcome of your pregnancy depends on keeping blood sugar near normal after meals. Your insulin needs change radically from one trimester to the next, and your meal plan will need to be adjusted to the changing demands on your body of the growing fetus. This is the time when you need to be in very close touch with your diabetes doctor, obstetrician, dietitian, and diabetes educator, if possible.

A natural question is: Will my hypoglycemic episodes affect my baby? The published research reports have been reassuring. If you treat hypoglycemia promptly, you and the baby recover quickly.

The new mom

After your baby is born, you should return to your pre-pregnancy insulin levels and meal plan—unless you are breastfeeding. Breastfeeding provides your child with the best nourishment and protection with antibodies from your body. Most children benefit greatly from even a few months of breastfeeding. If you breastfeed your baby, you need to see your dietitian to develop a meal plan with enough calories to nourish you and the baby and enough carbohydrate in meals and snacks to prevent hypoglycemia when you are nursing or in the middle of the night or at any time.

Whether you breastfeed or not, you must be very careful to eat and take your insulin on time, even though the demands on your time have increased. You cannot take good care of your baby if you don't take good care of yourself first.

Always keep a snack close by to avoid going too low while you're caring for the baby.

Plan ahead

Planning a pregnancy makes good sense for any couple, but when the woman has diabetes, it is much more important. Getting your diabetes under careful control before trying to get pregnant is strongly recommended. You'll learn much as you establish good control that will make controlling diabetes during pregnancy easier.

12

While You Sleep

Most severe episodes of hypoglycemia occur while you are sleeping. During such episodes, we are unable to take care of ourselves. We cannot feed ourselves and often resist relatives who try to feed us. On many occasions, we may be having convulsions or at least spastic jerking of the body and may even be deeply unconscious. We may have no control of what we are doing and often have little or no memory of what happened after we recover.

When you consider that episodes of severe hypoglycemia are remarkably common, you should try hard to avoid them or have someone nearby who will treat them aggressively. More than 10% of people who have type 1 diabetes will have had a severe episode within the past year, and 3% have recurrent episodes. In the DCCT (page 11), among the patients who were being treated in the conventional manner—not with tight control—10% had at least one episode of severe hypoglycemia during the first year of the study. In the tight control group, 26% had such an episode. We don't know how often severe hypoglycemia happens because most episodes are treated by relatives at home, and even if they report it to the doctor, the information is not collected or published.

If a severe insulin reaction occurs when you are sleeping alone, you may not recover because you may not get any treatment at all! Fortunately, in most cases if the insulin excess is not too severe, the body's counter-regulatory hormones and alternate sources of energy for the brain, such as fatty acids, come into play and the person survives. In many cases, some friends, relatives, or work associates wonder why the person didn't appear for breakfast, for work, for an appointment, or for school and call. When no one answers the phone, they begin to get worried. Since many of these people know that the person has diabetes and may even know that he or she is subject to insulin reactions, they quickly investigate. These people may find the person unconscious and call an ambulance to take him or her to an emergency room.

Diabetics who sleep alone in a motel or hotel room while traveling and have a severe hypoglycemic episode may be found by the hotel maid. Once while traveling alone, Dr. Lincoln failed to appear for breakfast. His associates came to his room, pounded on the door and were able to arouse him enough so that he could feed himself some candy. He recovered quickly, but it was a close call (chapter 14).

Children with Diabetes

Parents of children with type 1 diabetes who have experienced the problem of getting their child to eat during a severe hypoglycemic episode wonder if they should have the child sleep in their bedroom, so they would be awakened more quickly. With children less than 5 years old, such an arrangement may be okay, but the older children get, the more important privacy is to them and to parents. An adolescent doesn't usually mind sleeping in a room with a sibling, but sleeping in the same room with her parents would be highly unacceptable.

If your child sleeps in a separate room, how will you know that a severe insulin reaction is occurring? On many occasions, the child will cry out, groan, or breathe loudly and thrash about in the bed enough to wake the parents. Sometimes the child or adolescent will get out of bed in an agitated or confused state and knock down a lamp or a piece of furniture and wake the household. The child may be sufficiently alert to realize that he needs to eat and will go to the refrigerator to get something to eat. But the effort required to get to the refrigerator may be just enough to cause him to collapse or even fall downstairs.

When your children or adolescents go for overnight visits to relatives or friends, it is important that someone in that household knows what needs to be done if the child has a severe low blood sugar at night. Children and adolescents are extremely anxious to appear as normal as possible, so when you discuss what to do with your relatives or the parents, be private and don't exaggerate the risks. It is better for them to be aware ahead of time what might happen and to learn how to handle the episode. The same problem exists when children and adolescents are allowed to go on school trips where they will be staying overnight. Because fellow students cannot be expected to handle severe hypoglycemia in another child, you, a teacher, or experienced friend should watch out for the child.

What Your Adult Children Can Do For You

When you are sleeping at home alone, your children should call you in the morning to be sure that you are all right. We know of children who have called the telephone operator and pleaded for help when their mother had a severe insulin reaction. Most know to seek help from the neighbors or call a relative or friend who can go check on the parent. When you sleep alone and no one else is in the house, the risk of a severe hypoglycemic episode going undetected is considerable. The risk is greater when most of your neighbors work and are not at home during the day.

Once most people have experienced a severe hypoglycemic episode, they generally will be more careful in the future. Some people, however, learn slowly and do not seem to appreciate that another severe hypoglycemic episode is likely to happen sometime. It is wise to be prepared for another episode. In spite of this logic, it is surprising how many people and their families make the same mistakes over and over again.

Be Prepared

If you are sleeping alone, either at home or away, always check your blood glucose before you go to bed. If it is less than 125 mg/dl, you should have a small snack. The amount would depend on the type of insulin you took both in the morning and in the evening and the amount of exercise you had during the day. When sleeping alone at home, you may need to allow your blood glucose to go a little higher than normal. Ways to prevent hypoglycemia while sleeping alone are given in Table 12-1.

People who use NPH or lente insulin before their evening meal must remember that these types of insulin tend to have peak activity between 6 and 10 hours after the injection. If you keep having hypoglycemia in the early morning hours, and you cannot prevent it with a bedtime snack, then

TABLE 12-1

Ways to Prevent Hypoglycemia While Sleeping

1. Test your blood glucose before going to bed.

2. Eat a snack at bedtime.

3. Set an alarm clock to wake you up during the night to check on your condition.

4. Arrange to call a friend or relative each morning so that your friend knows that you are okay.

5. Maintain good control of blood glucose during the day but relax control somewhat during the night.

you need a change in your insulin plan. If you use rapid-acting or short-acting insulin to correct high blood sugar, be very careful when you use either insulin at bedtime. Your target blood glucose during sleeping hours should be no less than 125 mg/dl. It is safer to have a higher blood glucose level during the night and correct it when you wake in the morning than to increase the risk of hypoglycemia during the hours of sleep.

You should always have some type of sweet drink or glucose at your bedside every night. Even if you are married and your spouse sleeps in the same bed with you, it is essential to have sweets within your easy reach. You may get up during the night when you have moderate hypoglycemia and go into the bathroom and get so confused that you can no longer get back to your bedside table. It is always wise to have another supply of sweets or glucose in the bathroom. Keep the sweets in the same location because you may be in no mental condition to open drawers and search for food.

You can also set an alarm clock to go off between 1:00 a.m. and 3:00 a.m. You can get up and check your blood glucose level or go to the bathroom and wake up enough to be sure you are not hypoglycemic. Many people do this even when their spouse is sleeping in the same bed. Bed partners often sleep soundly and may not wake when you start to have difficulty. After you have had a number of nighttime hypoglycemic episodes, you learn to be careful.

When you will be sleeping alone in a hotel room, a wise precaution is to call before 7:00 a.m. and assure your spouse that you got through the night okay. You can exchange messages and express love, so your spouse is sure that you are okay. Some of these precautions may seem burdensome, but they are a small price to pay to prevent the consequences of a severe episode of hypoglycemia when you sleep alone.

13

Driving or Flying Safely

Most people who have had type 1 diabetes for more than 10 years will have experienced at least one mild hypoglycemic episode while driving. Hypoglycemia can seriously impair alertness, delay reaction time, and interfere with your judgment. If you take insulin, you must be extremely careful when you drive to avoid accidents caused by low blood sugar. Here are three stories that are pretty typical of what can happen.

A retired mechanic tells about an accident that he had many years ago brought on by hypoglycemia. He had an urgent project with his union that required some writing. A meeting had been scheduled Saturday morning to finish a report. He took the normal amount of insulin and had his usual breakfast. He then walked quite briskly for three miles to get some exercise. Without eating anything more, he got into his car and drove for about ten miles to reach the meeting place. His union group worked very hard on the report for 2 to 3 hours and during that time he did not eat anything. He said that his associates later thought that he had been functioning normally.

He was anxious to get back home, so he got into his car about 11:00 a.m. and started home. He drove off the road and bounced off several rock piles in a quarry and then stopped with the front end of his car hanging off the edge of a rock shelf. It was a miracle that it didn't go all the way into the pond below the shelf. The car was "totaled." He was taken to the hospital and given intravenous glucose and recovered immediately. He doesn't remember what happened or that he drove off the highway. The local newspaper wrote a big story, and he missed several days work because of soreness. He was extremely embarrassed and depressed for many days because of his carelessness. He was thankful that no one else was involved in the accident.

A middle-aged receptionist tells about her hypoglycemic driving accident. She got up one morning at her usual time and took her insulin injection in her arm. "I must have given myself too much insulin. I had my usual breakfast, but I didn't feel quite right when I left for work. I drove across a busy highway and got lost. I continued driving and felt weaker and weaker." One of her friends found her sitting at a red light. The car was not running. It was not at a very busy intersection so apparently other cars could get around her. The friend rolled down his window and said, "I have to get my wife to work. I'll be back in a minute and help you." He apparently thought her problem was "car trouble" and drove off. Then our low blood sugar lady started up her car, drove down the highway, and eventually off the road. "I wrecked it. I totaled it. I broke my nose and had lacerations on my hands. My neck was broken. No other car was involved." When she "came to" at the hospital after receiving some intravenous glucose, her first concern was, "Did I hurt anybody else?"

A middle-aged sales professional tells how he had his hypoglycemic accident many years ago. "I was going down the road, and I thought I saw four or five cars cross the road. I swerved to the left and gave it some gas like I was a football player. I hit the left rear fender of a car on the road. The jolt brought me out of it. This lady had parked at a beauty shop. Instead of parking in the parking lot, she had parked on the road. She came running out. I got out of my car and went into a little store and got me a Coke. I knew she thought I didn't care. Back then I didn't carry any sweets in the car. I got out of the mess by paying for the damages, but I was sure embarrassed. I later carried bottled Cokes. They got hot, but I could still drink them if my sugar got too low. I have also carried LifeSavers because they don't melt when the car gets hot during the summer."

In many accidents, the driver has obviously been hypoglycemic for some time and was seen swerving back and forth on the highway. It is likely that many of the hypoglycemic drivers had an inkling that they were getting low or at least were not feeling completely normal. What is most disturbing is that they continued to drive until they had a serious accident.

We would like for you to learn from their mistakes and not let your low blood sugar cause an accident. It is essential to check your blood sugar before you drive. We know that's not always possible or practical, but you can always, always, always have food or soda or a juice box in your car. It may be wise to eat a snack before you start.

If you have been sitting and watching a movie or attending church, you may not be aware that you are developing hypoglycemia. You leave the theater or church and get into your car and assume that you are okay. When you get into heavy traffic, you may suddenly realize that you are not okay. Your typical reaction is to tense up and "hold on" until you can get something to eat or you can get off the roadway. Too often your reaction is, "I guess I am a little low, but I don't have far to go. I'll eat as soon as I get home." Don't wait. Drink the juice you always carry in your car.

Often, after a close call or an accident, drivers with diabetes will admit privately that they were getting "low" but seemed to have almost a compulsion to continue driving. They knew better but just didn't want to bother to stop and just didn't want to do anything but keep on driving. Even your spouse may not be able to get you to stop and eat. Please be aware of your responsibility and don't let it get to this point.

Advice for Drivers with Diabetes

You should always have some form of candy available either in your pocket, in your purse, or somewhere on the seat or between the front seats within easy reach. Food stored in the glove compartment in the car is not within easy reach! Too often it will be lost under maps and papers. Fumbling around for candy while still trying to drive can be dangerous for any driver.

Unless you have just eaten or have determined your blood glucose level to be safe, eat some carbohydrate before you drive. Until you have a close call, you will probably ignore this piece of advice. Popping a piece of candy into your mouth at the same time as turning the key in the ignition can be a life saving routine. It should be as automatic as being sure you have your driver's license. If your snacking causes your blood glucose to rise too much, you can get it down later. Driving safely is more important than maintaining ideal blood glucose! (See Table 13-1.)

Know the times of day when you are most vulnerable to hypoglycemia. For example, patients on NPH or lente insulin usually have their lowest blood glucose about 8–12 hours after the injection. Generally, just before meals is also a time to be especially careful. If Dr. Lincoln's wife is with him, she won't let him drive before meals!

Consuming alcoholic beverages before driving is even more hazardous for people with diabetes. Even if you have had only a small quantity of alcohol, it can diminish your awareness of the early symptoms of hypoglycemia. This combination can be disastrous.

To avoid being falsely accused of intoxication, always wear a diabetes identification bracelet or necklace. If you should be seriously injured, it is extremely important that emergency room and ambulance attendants find out that you have diabetes as quickly as possible. Unfortunately, many times the importance of wearing such diabetes identification jewelry doesn't become apparent until after a dangerously close call. If you will accept the experiences of hundreds of people with diabetes, you'll get such jewelry and wear it.

Avoid any medication that could cause sedation. You need all the alertness that you can possibly maintain to recognize developing hypoglycemia. Many cold and allergy over-the-counter medicines cause sleepiness or diminished alertness. Reduced alertness might not be dangerous in usual daily activities but when you are driving long distances, it can be. If lack of awareness ever becomes a major problem for you, check your blood glucose before starting to drive and then every 2 to 3 hours to be sure you have adequate blood glucose to remain alert.

Long trips

Driving on long trips of 200 or more miles without stopping can be especially hazardous. The interstate highway, with its two lanes each way, no stop lights, no sharp turns, no cars or

TABLE 13-1

Tips for Safe Driving

1. Always have candy within easy reach in your car.

2. Eat something before you drive and snack periodically during long drives.

3. Know the times of the day when you are most vulnerable to hypoglycemia.

4. Don't drive alone on long trips.

5. On long trips, tell your passengers that you are a diabetic.

6. If you have drunk any alcoholic beverage, don't drive.

7. Always wear diabetes identification jewelry.

8. Avoid medications that sedate or make you sleepy.

9. Be especially careful after attending movies, concerts and church services.

10. If you have lost awareness of hypoglycemia symptoms, check your blood glucose before you drive and every 2–3 hours on long trips.

trucks suddenly entering from the side, and relatively low traffic volume, causes you to relax instead of being alert. Your blood sugar can drop gradually, and you and the other passengers in the car may not realize it.

Our advice is: Don't drive alone on a long trip. Although never driving alone on a long trip may seem to be much too restrictive, it is something you should avoid. As you get fatigued during driving, it is much easier to miss the subtle signals of early hypoglycemia. If you are careful to stop every 100–150 miles to measure your blood glucose, then the risk might be tolerable.

On long trips, tell your passengers that you have diabetes and may need to have periodic snacks. The fact that you made this admission will be reassuring to your passengers. It also makes it easier for you to admit to yourself and your passengers that you need to eat. Some people can be embarrassed by not having enough of their candy to pass around to everybody else in the car. If the passengers know that you are eating candy to meet a specific medical need, there should be no embarrassment.

Getting a driver's license

Commercial vehicles. Only nine states prevent people who use insulin from getting a commercial motor vehicle (CMV) operator's license. A CMV is usually a truck or bus weighing more than five tons that is engaged in business activity. In April 1992, licensing requirements of CMV drivers who travel across state boundaries were standardized to the Federal Highway Administration (FHA) guidelines. These guidelines require drivers who use insulin to have a medical examination every 6 months and to keep a log of blood glucose levels every 4 hours while driving.

Although the federal standard allows people using insulin to become CMV drivers, the restrictions discourage many from applying for a license. The European Community (EC) does not allow insulin-treated commercial drivers. When people with diabetes want to get or renew a CMV license, physicians carefully evaluate their diabetes control. These drivers may drive thousands of miles each year, often under bad weather or traffic conditions and often for many hours without rest. A CMV driver who drives across state boundaries must comply with federal regulations.

Private vehicles. Getting a private driver's license for most people with diabetes is seldom a problem. Many people don't bother to admit that they have diabetes when they apply for a driver's license. However, you may jeopardize your insurance if you have an accident and had failed to report your diabetes when you applied for a license or insurance. In many states, once you have a driver's license, you don't have to renew it for many years. If you were diagnosed with diabetes in the meantime, you need to report it. When you go to renew, you'll probably need a written statement from your physician that your diabetes is under good control. Your doctor wants to help you keep your driving privileges; however, if an accident occurs, the physician may be held partly to blame. Accept your responsibility to drive safely.

A major concern is that if physicians are required to report medical conditions of their patients to the police or licensing authorities, patients will withhold information. Any time you can't be comfortable describing your experiences of hypoglycemia to your physician, you may just not tell. When that happens, you have lost a valuable opportunity to learn more from your physician about controlling your blood glucose.

In recent years, there have been cases of drivers being sued for negligence for driving when they were physically impaired and causing an accident. In turn, some drivers sue their physicians for not having adequately informed them about the risks of driving or the precautions they should have taken. In one case, a person with diabetes was found guilty of failing to keep chocolate or sugar on hand to offset the effects of possible hypoglycemia while driving. In a case where the physician was being sued, the judge said, "it is as much a part of the professional duty to give correct information on the character of the disease from which the patient is suffering as it is to make a correct diagnosis or to prescribe appropriate medicine."

We tell you about these legal pressures as a warning to you and your physician. A major accident that results in death or injuries to several people caused by hypoglycemia could bring media pressure for more stringent regulations of diabetic drivers. Requirements for more thorough accident investigation and more detailed physician reporting could be the result. All of us need to realize that we have a personal responsibility to all other diabetic drivers. Regulations that would prevent us from getting a driver's license would be a severe handicap for us all.

Flying an Airplane

Until recently, people with diabetes could not get a license to fly. The long-standing rule was that anyone who had an established history or clinical diagnosis of diabetes that requires insulin or any other hypoglycemic drug for control would not be allowed to take the pilots' examination.

The Federal Aviation Administration (FAA) now permits pilots with diabetes to hold a third-class medical certification. This allows you to be a private, recreational, or student pilot. An airline transport pilot holds a first-class medical certificate. Glider and free balloon pilots are not required to hold a medical certificate of any class. There are several conditions that you must meet to earn the medical certification to fly.

1. You must have had no recurrent (two or more) episodes of hypoglycemia in the past 5 years and none in the preceding year resulting in a loss of consciousness, seizure, impaired cognitive function, or requiring intervention by another person, or that occurred without warning (hypoglycemia unawareness). Cognitive function means the mental activities associated with think-

ing, learning, and memory—in other words, alertness
and clear thinking.
2. The applicant is required to provide copies of all perti-
nent medical records.
3. A report of a complete medical examination is required, which must include the following:
   a. Two measurements of HbA1c, one at least 90 days
   prior to a current measurement (chapter 4).
   b. The insulin dose and the meal plan.
   c. The presence or absence of any cardiovascular disease or neuropathy.
   d. The absence of clinically significant eye disease
   (retinopathy).
   e. Verification that the applicant has been educated in
   the importance of control of diabetes and "under-
   stands the actions that should be taken if complications, especially hypoglycemia, should arise."
   f. If the applicant is age 40 or older, a report of a maxi-
   mal exercise stress test to detect early coronary heart
   disease must be provided with the ECG tracings.
   g. The applicant must be able to determine blood glucose levels using a recording glucometer.

The protocol requires you to have a detailed physical
exam. With the present emphasis on maintaining near normal
blood glucose, it is difficult for anyone to say that they have
not had any episodes of severe hypoglycemia. You might be
tempted to stretch the truth, but we ask you to think about
the situations that could develop. Just as with driving, there
are long stretches when flying is not difficult, and you may
not realize that your blood sugar is dropping and affecting
your ability to react quickly and do what you need to do.
During landing and taking off, as well as around busy airports

or in poor weather, you need to be alert and working well. Even if you eat immediately, it still takes 10–15 minutes before your alertness returns. If you have forgotten to bring anything to eat with you, it could be 15 minutes to an hour before you can land and get something to eat.

When you fly, check your blood glucose every hour, and always have some glucose tablets or food near you on the plane to eat if you realize that you are developing hypoglycemia.

Whether you are driving or flying, or even riding a bicycle, people who live with diabetes should accept the Boy Scout motto and always "Be Prepared" for hypoglycemia.

14

Traveling and Hypoglycemia

You can travel to any location but there are many precautions that are necessary. You like to assume that everything will go just as you have planned, but you have to be prepared for a disruption of your travel plans. Meals may not be on time, menu choices may be limited, opportunities for exercise could be greatly reduced, and support people like family, friends, or work associates may not be available to help you. Your luggage may get lost, and you may not be able to get into the hotel where you had a reservation. Many times you will be completely alone when you sleep at night.

Dr. Lincoln has traveled all over the world and has had to adjust to some difficult situations. He never had any serious episodes of hypoglycemia while traveling until a memorable episode about 10 years ago.

He says: I was on a business trip to Allentown, PA, and had to make a change in Pittsburgh. I boarded my plane in Knoxville, TN, at about 11:30 a.m. I had expected to be given a snack, but I had not taken my before-meal dose of regular insulin so was not overly concerned when the snack was not served. I was sleepy, so I pushed back my seat and took a nap.

I awakened as the plane landed. I don't remember what shape I was in, but I got off the plane and walked toward my next gate. I don't know how far I walked but I remember that I suddenly realized that I had left my carry-on bag on the airplane. I turned around and started almost running to go back to the gate from which I had come.

The next thing I knew, I was waking up in a local hospital emergency room. I had collapsed in the airport concourse and was picked up by emergency medical technicians and transported by ambulance to a nearby hospital. The airport supervisor had gotten my home telephone number out of my wallet and called my wife. She was told that I was unconscious, and they thought I had probably had a heart attack. She immediately told the supervisor that I was a diabetic and was probably having an insulin reaction. He said he would radio that information to the ambulance and the hospital. Soon after I arrived at the emergency room, I was given glucose intravenously, and I recovered quickly. I had to struggle a bit to convince the ER physicians that I was okay. I needed to get back to the airport to catch the next flight to Allentown. I was soon released and hitched a ride to the airport with an ambulance crew. My carry-on bag had gone on to Baltimore but was quickly found, and I was able to get it at the Allentown airport by 10:00 p.m.

This episode taught me never to sleep on an airplane if I am alone unless I know that my blood glucose is okay. Also, when I realized that I was going to miss a meal, I should have checked my blood glucose to see what my level was and then eaten enough candy or asked for a regular Coke to be sure I would not get too low. I should have had a wrist bracelet or necklace identifying me as having diabetes. These were three mistakes in a physician with diabetes who should have known better! I had been careless because I assumed that nothing would ever happen to me.

One of the greatest dangers of traveling alone is when you are sleeping. Frequently, your usual eating patterns have been disrupted and your blood glucose level at bedtime may not have quite the same meaning as it does at home. If you have gone to a banquet, your blood glucose at bedtime may be unusually high, and in order to get to sleep you might take some extra rapid-acting insulin. If you took extra insulin before the banquet and then found that your glucose was low at bedtime, you may have difficulty getting the same snack that you normally use at bedtime at home. You will have to improvise using candy, cookies, or sugary beverages that you can purchase from a vending machine.

When you travel long distances across several time zones, your insulin and eating schedule get disrupted. If you travel from the Eastern Time Zone to the west coast, the intermediate-acting insulin that you took in the morning before you left will still be functioning on your home time. It will be three hours earlier on Pacific Time, so you may not feel that you need to eat until 6:00 p.m. local time. Your insulin schedule requires you to eat at 3:00 p.m.

If you live on the west coast and travel east and you take your intermediate insulin at 7:00 a.m. Pacific Time, it will be 3:00 p.m. in California when it is dinner time (by the clock) in the East. Your risk is less when you are going east, but eating early may cause your blood glucose at bedtime to be higher than expected.

There are several important precautions that you should think through before leaving on a long trip alone. These are summarized in Table 14-1. If you can, try to plan a flexible schedule. Allow yourself extra time for eating and for traveling to and from the airport. When you are pressed for time, it is much easier to make mistakes in judgment regarding your blood glucose and your need to eat.

TABLE 14-1

Travel Checklist

1. Have some flexibility in your schedule.

2. Always wear a medical ID bracelet or necklace.

3. Carry insulin, meter, and food with you at all times.

4. Check your blood glucose level more frequently when traveling.

5. During a flight, wait to take your rapid-acting insulin until your meal has been served.

6. Always take your own alarm clock.

7. Have something sweet on your bedside table as well as in the bathroom.

8. Call your spouse or family in the morning so that they know you are okay.

9. Keep your family and business associates informed of your travel plans.

10. Let the hotel clerk know that you have diabetes.

Always wear an identification bracelet or necklace stating that you have diabetes, and be sure that you have a card in your wallet or purse that identifies you as a diabetic who takes insulin. Be sure that your card gives your closest relative's telephone number and at least two other numbers of friends, relatives, or work associates who could be called if no one answers at the first number.

Always carry more than enough insulin, testing supplies, and food in your carry-on bag and candy or glucose tablets in your pocket or purse so that you can survive at least 24 hours even if you lose all your luggage. Don't worry about refrigeration of the insulin. It is remarkably stable, and several days at room temperature will not significantly impair its effectiveness. Check your blood glucose more frequently, so you know better what your blood glucose level is. Don't depend on how you feel. Awareness of developing hypoglycemia is frequently impaired during travel.

If you take rapid-acting insulin before a meal, wait until you are being served. If you can't get into the airplane rest room to take your insulin, you can do it in your seat. Just explain to your seat neighbor that you have diabetes and need to take insulin before you eat. Many times there can be long delays in being served. If you have taken your insulin and sudden turbulence requires the crew to stop serving a meal, you will need to eat some of the candy that you carry with you.

Although most hotels have alarm clocks in their rooms, you should always carry your own clock. Set the alarm to go off 3–4 hours after you go to bed, so you will wake up and determine if you are okay. As a precaution, the clock should be placed as far on the other side of the bedside table as possible so you won't reach over and shut it off and go back to sleep. As a further precaution, get up and go to the bathroom and if necessary, check your blood glucose. If you are low, avoid drinking beverages that have caffeine in them or you may have difficulty getting back to sleep.

As a precaution, have something sweet that is easy to eat or drink both on your bedside table and in the bathroom. If you should get up with low blood glucose and stagger into the bathroom, you need to have something there to eat. You might not be able to make it back to the bedside table.

Before traveling alone, practice eating out at irregular times so you learn how to adjust your eating and insulin schedule. There are no easy formulas. Experience is your best teacher. Always keep your family and work associates informed about any changes in your travel plans.

It is a good idea to let the hotel personnel know that you have diabetes. Most hotels have had experience with patrons having severe hypoglycemic episodes during the night and will ask you to advise them in the morning that you got through the night okay.

Be aware that when you are traveling, especially on vacation, you may walk and get more exercise than you usually do. This will lower your blood glucose more than you expect into the night and the next day, when you'll be walking again. Take care to check your blood glucose often and always have candy or glucose tablets with you.

15

Alcohol and Hypoglycemia

Y ou can enjoy an occasional glass of wine. However, alcohol can interfere with management of your diabetes and cause you to miss the symptoms of dropping blood glucose. Table 15-1 lists 12 reasons you should be conservative in the amount of alcohol that you drink.

It is easy to forget or maybe not even think about the caloric content of alcohol. Each gram of alcohol furnishes 7 calories, while carbohydrates and protein have only 4 calories per gram. The calories associated with alcohol are "empty" calories. They do not provide anything that the body needs. When too much alcohol (especially beer) is consumed over long periods of time, obesity is a common result.

Alcohol dulls alertness. This is called relaxation or loss of inhibition and is probably the major reason why many people enjoy an occasional cocktail, a glass of wine, or a can of beer. Alcohol is a social lubricant. It gets people to talk and smile and forget about their worries. Unfortunately, alcohol also diminishes awareness of your early symptoms of hypoglycemia.

Sometimes you may take insulin or your diabetes pills assuming that a meal will be served on time or that the

TABLE 15-1

The Dangers of Alcohol

1. Diminishes your awareness of the symptoms of hypoglycemia

2. Increases the risk of hypoglycemia

3. Is toxic to nerves and may aggravate diabetic neuropathy

4. May impair sexual performance

5. Increases high blood pressure

6. May aggravate diabetic eye disease

7. Raises level of triglycerides in blood, which may aggravate arteriosclerosis

8. Is metabolized like fat and adds to body weight

9. Delays recovery from hypoglycemia

10. Lowers motivation to maintain diabetes control

11. Diminishes the effectiveness of glucagon in treating severe hypoglycemia

12. Can prevent recovery from severe hypoglycemia and lead to death

appetizers before the meal will provide you enough calories to prevent any hypoglycemia from developing. When you are under the relaxing effect of alcohol, a delay in eating seems less important. Because conversations during a cocktail party are often light, you may not be aware that you are not thinking very clearly. Neither you nor your friends are as likely to notice that something other than alcohol is affecting you. The spouse who is usually extremely sensitive to changes in the husband's or wife's behavior may also miss the beginning signs of trouble.

The problem is determining how much of the behavior change is due to alcohol and how much is due to hypoglycemia. Do you always measure the quantity of alcohol you consume? Your dizziness could be hypoglycemia. Inappropriate answers just bounce off friends with a laugh. Other symptoms of hypoglycemia, especially sweating, are also easily ignored because rooms are often crowded and warm during parties.

Dr. Lincoln remembers two such occasions: It was warm in the room and there were many people milling about. The sweat poured off my brow, and I could feel my shirt getting soaked. I didn't think that I was hypoglycemic. I was talking and joking and having a good time. But I was embarrassed by having to mop the sweat off my face and bald head with my handkerchief. I complained to others that the room seemed to be unusually warm, but they hadn't noticed it and were not complaining. My wife was not with me, so she couldn't get me to eat something sweet. I began to notice that I was not relating very well to people, and I had a vague uneasiness. I finally realized that I was getting into trouble and fled to a rest room where I ate numerous M&M candies until I recovered. I went back to the party with a dry head but with a soaked shirt and severely dampened suit and was uncomfortable the rest of the evening.

On another occasion, it appeared to my wife that I was becoming unusually quiet and withdrawn. I didn't seem to recognize people I should have known well. She whispered to me, "Honey, you need to eat." I reacted like most diabetics who are mildly hypoglycemic, "I'm all right! I don't need to eat! Leave me alone!" She, being the caring wife she is, persisted. She knew that if I didn't get something to eat, I would rapidly get worse and might make a fool of myself. I was irritated because she was nagging me in public and other people might see us arguing. The more she pushed the more irritated I got.

Finally, she went to the table and got some sweets. She said, "Here, honey, I think this will help." I ate and in a few minutes, was back to normal. I realized that I had started to have difficulty about 20 minutes earlier. As I have long realized, my wife is always right. I don't know how long it would have been before I recognized what the real problem was, but only a few minutes could have been too long. I'm sure that you, like me, want to avoid the embarrassment of having low blood sugar at a party.

The brain constitutes only 2% of body weight, but it requires more than 50% of the glucose output of the liver. The hypoglycemic action of alcohol adds to that of insulin and may cause such severe hypoglycemia that neurological damage can result. This is why you should always eat food when you are having a drink.

When you have mild hypoglycemia after having one or two drinks, it can be treated the same way as when you are not drinking. The best foods to eat are sweetened carbonated beverages or fruit juices (chapter 5). Cheese and crackers or other appetizers take longer to eat and to digest, so they raise your blood glucose much more slowly. A person who is severely hypoglycemic but is also intoxicated with alcohol has to be aggressively treated. Because glycogen stores in the liver are already reduced, glucagon treatment may not be as effective. This individual should be taken to an emergency room at a hospital and given intravenous glucose.

People who consume a lot of alcoholic beverages as a habit seldom have good control of their diabetes. When hypoglycemia and intoxication occur together, people with diabetes run a great danger of total collapse. Other people will probably regard them as being drunk and often will not make an effort to help them. Hypoglycemia without any alcohol consumption often looks like drunkenness. It can be difficult to tell them apart.

If you have had diabetes for many years, you may have lost much of your early awareness of developing hypoglycemia (chapter 19). The symptoms of jitteriness, shaking, profuse perspiration, hunger, and rapid pulse tend to disappear or, at least, to become less prominent. As a consequence, you have to depend on subtle changes in mental function or changes in your behavior to alert you to hypoglycemia. These subtle changes are much less apparent when you have had a drink or two. Of course, when there is doubt, you can check your blood glucose and get information about your condition.

If you have had a couple drinks and are suspicious that you may be developing hypoglycemia, don't try to hold out until a meal is served. Eating times at parties are very hard to predict. If you have eaten some hors d'ouevres and think that you can wait until they have been digested, you may get into trouble. Symptoms of hypoglycemia depend only on what the level of glucose is in the brain at a specific moment. Your blood glucose may be rising slowly but until it gets above about 60 mg/dl, your hypoglycemic symptoms can still be a serious problem. During that few minutes of waiting, you can make a fool of yourself and regret it for months or years. When in the slightest doubt, drink a sweet cola as a wise precaution.

Alcohol and complications

Alcohol can aggravate some of the complications of diabetes. Alcohol consumption, even in moderation, can worsen diabetic eye and nerve disease. Heavy alcohol consumption may increase the likelihood of leaking blood vessels in the retina of the eye and could lead to blindness. Alcohol in more than moderate amounts aggravates hypertension (high blood pressure). It increases the level of triglycerides in the blood, which may accelerate the deposits of fat in your arteries.

A study at the Harvard Medical School claimed to show that the risk of having a heart attack in people without diabetes was reduced when they regularly drank a glass of red wine. There was an increase in the amount of the good cholesterol (high-density lipoproteins [HDL]). People with diabetes are already more likely to have coronary heart disease and may feel that they now have justification to drink more. Please remember that you have special risks from alcohol and should not use this study and others as a justification to drink more alcohol.

16

Prescription Drugs and Hypoglycemia

Whenever you visit any medical facility, regardless of the reason, tell the physician that you have diabetes. Don't assume that the physician will always ask you. If you are being treated for something unrelated to your diabetes, it may not occur to the doctor to ask this question. If a prescription is given to you, always ask whether it will have any effect on your diabetes control.

Have an up-to-date list of all the medications you are taking and the dosage schedule in your wallet or pocketbook. If you are involved in an accident or suddenly taken ill, it can be of great value for emergency physicians to be able to learn quickly what medications you are taking. Remember that you may not be able to tell the physician yourself because you may be too ill or injured. Your spouse cannot be expected to remember exactly what medicines you are taking. Unless you have the actual pills with you, it is impossible for physicians or nurses to identify most medications on the basis of your description of their size, shape, or color.

Some common drugs prescribed for other conditions can cause or aggravate hypoglycemia. The oral drugs that are prescribed for type 2 diabetes can cause serious hypoglycemia. When this happens, it is usually because they have been improperly dispensed or wrongly used, or they interact with another drug. Some general rules, if followed, will greatly reduce the number of cases of hypoglycemia involving medications. They are summarized in Table 16-1.

At the Pharmacy

When you consider the millions of prescriptions that are filled each day, it is not surprising that mistakes in dispensing dia-

TABLE 16-1

Ways to Prevent Hypoglycemia from Medications

1. Keep diabetes pills separate from all other medications.

2. Containers of diabetes pills should be marked with colored tape so recognition is easier.

3. Wrap colored or sticky tape around the neck of NPH or ultralente insulin bottles, so you won't confuse them with bottles of regular or rapid-acting insulin.

4. Tell all physicians that you have diabetes regardless of the reason for your medical visit.

5. Be extremely careful if you start a diet while taking diabetes pills or insulin.

6. Have an up-to-date list of all your medications in your wallet or purse.

7. Many medications greatly decrease your awareness of hypoglycemic symptoms. Ask your physician how any drug prescribed will affect your blood glucose level.

8. Like alcohol, many illegal drugs reduce awareness of hypoglycemia and prevent you from taking action.

betes medications occasionally occur. Chlorpromazine (Thorazine), a medication used to treat schizophrenia, has been confused with chlorpropamide (Diabenese), used in treating type 2 diabetes. As you can see, the generic names are quite similar. Tablets of chlorpropamide have been dispensed and labeled as chloroquine, a drug used to treat malaria and to treat arthritis. Tablets of glyburide (DiaBeta), a type 2 drug, have been dispensed instead of lorazepam (a tranquilizer). Because these blood glucose–lowering medications sometimes interact with other prescription medications, cases of severe hypoglycemia have occurred. Check the label and/or the pills before leaving the pharmacy.

An example of a different type of interaction is the effect of propranolol. This medication is used to treat hypertension, angina of coronary heart disease, and rhythm disturbances in several other types of heart disease. A side effect discovered by actors using it for heart disease was the calming effect it had on their stage fright. It was soon prescribed for patients who had anxiety. Some of these patients had diabetes, and it was discovered that this medication caused a reduction of their awareness of hypoglycemia. Let your doctors know you have diabetes—even psychiatrists. Ask your pharmacist if any of your medications will affect your alertness to hypoglycemia.

At Home

Some people take different types of medicine on different schedules and get confused about how much they should take of each of their pills. Many mistakes occur when people forget that they have already taken their daily dose or think that their physician said to increase the amount. Sometimes this confusion persists and they may continue to take too many pills over a period of several days. It is even possible to confuse diabetes pills with artificial sweeteners. In one reported case, a woman put three glyburide tablets (an oral hypoglycemic medication) in her diabetic husband's oatmeal instead of an artificial sweetener!

The possible hypoglycemic effect of dieting is a major cause for concern. Patients taking diabetes pills sometimes decide to go on crash diets to try to lose weight. They don't reduce their medication for the smaller amount of food and often develop hypoglycemia. Early symptoms of hypoglycemia may be mistakenly interpreted as weakness due to dieting. Elderly patients are particularly vulnerable to the hypoglycemic effects of these diabetes medications.

In type 2 diabetes, hypoglycemia caused by diabetes pills often comes on slowly and is not recognized early by you or your family members. People with type 2 diabetes don't wear medical identification jewelry as often as do people with type 1. You may want to start wearing a medical ID now.

When low blood sugar occurs as a result of taking pills for diabetes, it is rarely as severe or as frequently low as when you use insulin. However, knowledge about the medicines and the potential for experiencing low blood sugar may help you minimize your risks.

There are currently three classes of diabetes pills for type 2 diabetes. Table 16-2 lists the medicines that stimulate the pancreas to release insulin. By increasing the amount of insulin circulating in your blood, any of these can cause hypoglycemia. If your blood sugar is close to normal and you take an overdose of these pills, skip a meal, or strenuously exercise, you are at risk of developing hypoglycemia. Note that some of these medications have long-lasting effects and can cause recurrent hypoglycemia until they are eliminated from the body. It is a wise and safe practice to check your blood sugar more

TABLE 16-2

Medications That Cause Release of Insulin

Generic name	Trade name	Duration of action (hours)
Tolazamide	Tolinase	10–14
Tolbutamide	Orinase	6–12
Chlorpropamide	Diabinese	72
Glyburide	Diabeta Micronase	18–24
Glipizide	Glucotrol	10–24
Glimeperide	Amaryl	18–28
Repaglinide	Prandin	3–5
Glyburide + Metformin	Glucovance	18–24

frequently when changing your dose or combining any of the medications that lower blood glucose.

Table 16-3 lists medications that reduce the amount of glucose released by the liver and reduce resistance to insulin by muscle and fat tissues. The drugs on this list do not cause hypoglycemia when you take just one kind of them. But if

TABLE 16-3

Medications That Reduce Insulin Resistance

Generic name	Trade name	Site of action
Pioglitizone	Actose	Muscle & Fat (Liver)
Rosiglitizone	Avandia	Muscle & Fat (Liver)
Metformin	Glucophage	Liver (Muscle & Fat)

TABLE 16-4

Medications That Slow the Absorption of Sugar

Generic name	Trade name	Site of action (hours)
Acarbose	Precose	Intestine/4
Miglitol	Glyset	Intestine/4

you also take insulin or one of the pills listed in Table 16-2, your blood glucose can go too low. You probably won't need as much insulin or as large a dose of the pills. Ask your doctor for guidance when combining any of the medications for diabetes. The medications listed in Table 16-3 reach full effect after 2–4 weeks of treatment, so be patient and cautious when adding them to your current treatment.

The third class of oral medicines slows down the absorption of sugars from the intestine following a meal (Table 16-4). These drugs must be taken just before eating a meal. They do not cause hypoglycemia when used alone. If the normal rise of blood sugar is prevented by these medications and you also use rapid-acting insulin, you can develop hypoglycemia within 1–2 hours. Always ask your doctor about how to safely begin when combining any medicines for your diabetes.

Most emergency physicians now routinely get a blood glucose level on every patient regardless of age who arrives at the hospital in a stupor or unconscious condition. They will do this test even when the cause of the condition may seem obvious, such as drunkenness, because many drugs can cause hypoglycemia, even in people who do not have diabetes. However, you can get taken care of much more quickly if they know you have diabetes. Are you wearing your medical ID?

Taking the wrong amount of insulin or diabetes pills is easier than most people realize. Sometimes you may be sleepy in the morning and forget to take your insulin or pill, or you may take it twice. If you take more than one type of insulin each day, you may measure out the wrong amount from one of your bottles. You may forget that you have already taken your insulin and take it a second time. Some people who take both regular and intermediate-acting insulin, such as NPH or lente, may, for example, take two injections of the longer-acting insulin rather than one of each. In such cases, the extra insulin would cause prolonged hypoglycemia. Better to mark one type of insulin with a piece of tape around the bottle or put a bright sticker on the label to remind you which is which. When your hypoglycemia is due to an overdose of oral hypoglycemic medicines, the hypoglycemia is much more difficult to treat and may require continuous intravenous glucose for many hours.

Mixed with other drugs

Sedatives, tranquilizers, sleeping tablets, antihistamines, or pain pills may decrease your awareness of approaching hypoglycemia. If you have to take any of these medications, use extreme care, especially if you have some difficulty recognizing the early signs of hypoglycemia. We don't mean that you cannot use these medications, but do remember the potential for problems.

You should be exceedingly careful about using sleeping pills. When sleep has been drug induced, you may not wake when you have signs of hypoglycemia. You may sink into deep unconsciousness before a spouse or family member recognizes that you are in serious trouble. As a general rule, don't take sedatives.

Although it should be obvious, using illegal drugs is extremely dangerous for you. These drugs affect the central nervous system and greatly reduce your awareness of hypoglycemia. They can also keep you from doing something to correct it. If you eat under the influence of the drugs, you may find that your blood glucose is much higher than normal, which will add to your stupor. This can get in the way of proper care at the emergency room, too.

17

The Effects of Hypoglycemia on Nerves and Vision

Motor nerves control our muscles, and sensory nerves inform us about the world around us. They may become impaired by hypoglycemia but usually only in a highly selective fashion. Hypoglycemia seldom seriously affects the peripheral nerves. The major problem occurs in the central nervous system or, more specifically, in the brain, which is exquisitely sensitive to a lack of glucose.

Certain brain functions may temporarily work poorly during hypoglycemia and cause alarming symptoms. They tend to last much longer than most symptoms of hypoglycemia. They may vary from widespread stroke-like effects to weakness in just one group of muscles. Convulsions or uncontrollable jerking motions of the body occur in 10–20% of adults and even more frequently in children when they have a severe hypoglycemic episode. It is important to be aware of some of these effects, so you won't panic if you should develop some of them. Your first impulse is to believe that permanent brain damage has occurred. What initially might be regarded as a stroke may turn out to be only a temporary problem. Complete return to normal may take a few hours to a few days.

Although episodes of hypoglycemia that initially look like a stroke are uncommon, they are not rare. Diabetes specialists have made note of them for over 50 years, and many cases have been reported in the medical literature.

A good example of a case of a presumed stroke was reported by Dr. Pell and Dr. Frier in Edinburgh, Scotland, in 1990. A 49-year-old man who had had diabetes for more than 30 years developed extreme muscle weakness on the right side of his body during a severe hypoglycemic episode. He had been comatose for about 2 hours when he was brought to the hospital. His blood glucose was only 20 mg/dl. He regained consciousness after being given intravenous glucose, but the muscular weakness continued. It gradually disappeared over the next month, and no cause other than the hypoglycemia could be found.

He later experienced further episodes of hypoglycemia and sometimes developed weakness. He learned that when he began to develop weakness and incoordination in his right hand, arm, and leg, he knew he was getting low. If he ate something quickly and got his blood glucose up, the weakness disappeared.

Many similar cases involving both younger and older people with diabetes have been reported. A 22-year-old man was brought to the hospital with total paralysis of his right side. His blood glucose was 40 mg/dl. A glucose solution was given intravenously, and the paralysis disappeared in less than 3 hours. He had another episode of right-side paralysis the next day during hypoglycemia, which rapidly disappeared when he was given glucose. This young man went on to have many more severe hypoglycemic episodes, but in the 3 years after the original episode, he never had any more paralysis.

Although generalized seizures can occur during severe hypoglycemia, they are uncommon. There may even be loss of bowel or bladder function during the seizure, but fortunately that is rare. Much more often, there are continuous muscle contractions, especially in the legs and arms. They look much like a convulsion, but the hypoglycemic patient can often still drink sweetened beverages poured into his mouth. He may not be unconscious and may even have a vivid memory of the muscular contractions after the hypoglycemia has been corrected. Since this type of severe hypoglycemia usually occurs at night, the next day he will complain that he feels "like I have been run over by a truck." The muscular soreness and general fatigue last 6–12 hours but then usually go away completely.

Older patients, especially women who have osteoporosis (thin bones due to loss of calcium), may get fractures in their spines during the seizure-like activity. Because of this, persistent pain and tenderness in bones or joints after a seizure need to be investigated.

The wife of a retired man who had taken insulin for 58 years described a sign that always alerted her to hypoglycemia in her husband. She noticed that when he seemed to have difficulty with his balance and needed to position his feet in a special way or hang on to a piece of furniture, she knew immediately that he was developing hypoglycemia. When his glucose was normal, he had no difficulty walking and standing.

If the problem clears promptly after you are given glucose, there has probably been no serious brain damage. But most diabetes specialists recommend several hours of observation after your severe hypoglycemia has been corrected. The neurologic problem may reappear if the hypoglycemia returns. If you have taken too much intermediate- or long-acting insulin or some of the diabetes pills that have long-lasting effects, your hypoglycemia may be long-lasting and difficult to treat.

A 4-year-old boy who had diabetes for 1 1/2 years walked into a pediatric clinic with his mother who said the boy had suddenly developed "crossed" eyes. The boy was alert but sweaty and had a rapid pulse. His blood glucose was 40 mg/dl. He ate a snack and within a few minutes his eyes uncrossed, and he could see perfectly normally. Two years later, he had the same sign during another episode of hypoglycemia.

Double vision is a fairly common symptom of hypo-glycemia. It is not initially associated with severe confusion, shakiness, or sweating. Dr. Eaddy has had several episodes of blurring of his vision. After he ate some sugar, the symptoms gradually disappeared over about 10–15 minutes. Double vision can be overcome temporarily by closing or covering one eye. If double vision should ever occur while you are driving, close one eye for the few minutes it takes you to safely stop and get something to eat.

Reading is frequently difficult during hypoglycemia. Most often it is due to a general dulling of brain function. You lose the ability to concentrate and understand what you are read-ing. Often there is difficulty following the lines of a manu-script. You may find that you have to constantly go back and reread lines in order to understand them.

Color vision is frequently impaired during hypoglycemia. If your color vision is already less than normal, the additional decline during hypoglycemia certainly has safety implications. If you didn't notice a color change, you could fail to correctly follow a traffic signal and have an accident.

Distant vision seems to be relatively unimpaired even dur-ing fairly severe hypoglycemia. The problem is in understand-ing what you are seeing. It isn't a good idea to go to an optometrist or ophthalmologist for an eye exam if you are even mildly hypoglycemic. You will have difficulty with the test, and you may be unhappy with the glasses you get.

People with diabetes who have poor control and consistently high blood glucose levels may also develop blurred vision. Indeed, vision problems are sometimes one of the early signs of developing diabetes. One of the degenerative complications of diabetes, called retinopathy, causes impaired vision, but it is not related to hypoglycemia. It is related to the prolonged high blood glucose levels associated with poor control of diabetes.

18

Psychological Insights

Those of us who live with insulin dependent diabetes frequently are confounded and frustrated by unanticipated hypoglycemia. These feelings are particularly strong when we are embarrassed, temporarily disabled, or made dependent on another person by our hypoglycemia. Dr. Eaddy says, "When I have taken special precautions using all of my knowledge and skill to manage my diabetes and I still have an insulin reaction, I get ANGRY!" The frustration and anger are real and need to be discussed.

Nearly everyone with diabetes will sooner or later have at least one hypoglycemic episode that will cause them deep personal embarrassment. Some will have many episodes. You may have acted like you were drunk and made a fool of yourself. You may have become irritable and said hateful things to your spouse or friends. You may have been unable to do some simple task and just acted silly. You may have just sat still, sweating like an exhausted boxer. You may have trembled while you babbled incoherently. You may have been unable to conduct a coherent conversation with your boss or teacher. You may have struck your wife or friend when they were trying to feed you. You may have run the lawn mower into your wife's garden of beautiful flowers.

Some people say they don't remember how they acted. Some will pass it off as a simple mistake in diabetes management. Most of you, however, will be deeply distressed after these public episodes. Your relatives and friends easily forgive you and give you generous sympathy. Nevertheless, each episode inflicts a psychological injury. Over a lifetime, these episodes will require you to adjust in many ways in order to thrive. In some cases, these episodes can cause serious psychological problems. This chapter touches briefly on some of these problems because we are concerned like you are, and we want to help you prevent problems or, at least, to view them realistically.

Handling Anger and Frustration

Feelings of frustration and anger are legitimate and appropriate when hypoglycemia still happens, no matter what precautions you have taken. Talking about those feelings with your family, friends, and health care providers helps reduce the intensity of the emotions that can interfere with the enjoyable parts of your life. Once the feelings are under control, it is a good idea to review the day's events to try to discover the cause of your hypoglycemia. Ask yourself questions, such as: Was the time or site of my insulin shot correct? What about heat, exercise, and depth of injection? Could I have injected improperly? If you can identify the cause, then there is hope that you can avoid a repeat episode. You can learn from your mistakes and avoid future unpleasant episodes of low blood sugar.

Episodes of hypoglycemia are going to occur if you are trying to achieve excellent blood sugar control. By measuring your blood glucose before each meal and at bedtime, keeping blood glucose records, and making notes that explain your highs and lows, you can learn to be in control of your diabetes most of the time. You can learn to make careful changes in your food choices, exercise plan, and insulin dose, if necessary, to reach your goal of blood sugar control. Have patience! Ask for advice from your team of diabetes advisors! Avoid over-reacting to isolated events of high or low blood sugar.

You must accept the fact that about 20% of the time, neither you nor your health care providers will know why your blood glucose is where it is. There are things in your life that are outside of your control. The present way we use insulin is only a simple attempt to mimic the action of a healthy pancreas. Despite your best efforts, there will be unpredictable hypoglycemic events. Let 'em go.

Self-induced hypoglycemia

Some people intentionally take too much insulin. The reason for taking so much insulin and having many severe hypoglycemic attacks may be related to some underlying psychological problem where they think they need sympathy. Patients who have frequent severe episodes of hypoglycemia sometimes claim that they are following exactly what their doctor told them to do. They steadfastly deny that they are taking more insulin than they were told to take. One patient studied at the National Institutes of Health in Bethesda, MD, admitted to self-administering up to 2,000 units of insulin per day! The psychiatric treatment of these people is often extremely difficult.

Brittle diabetes

Diabetes that has been described as brittle should not imply any kind of mental illness or behavioral disorder. Nevertheless, such patients experience much anxiety, frustration, and sometimes depression. Their families often have the same feelings.

Brittle diabetes has several definitions; a good one has been proposed by Professor Tattersall of the Department of Diabetes of the University Hospital in Nottingham, England. He said that the patient with brittle diabetes is one "whose life is constantly being disrupted by episodes of hypo or hyperglycemia, whatever their cause." He listed five causes (Table 18-1).

Errors of management are now largely avoidable by frequent home blood glucose monitoring and not overreacting to high or low blood glucose levels. Fear of eventual complications may cause patients or their families to give too much insulin when they have elevated blood glucose. That leads to low blood glucose, and then you need to eat extra food, which leads to high glucose. Then you need more insulin. The cycle is sometimes difficult to stop.

Most diabetic patients learn slowly not to overreact in their low glucose or high glucose adjustments. Brittle diabetes

---

TABLE 18-1

Causes of Brittle Diabetes

1. Errors of management
2. Excessive insulin dosage
3. Effects of other illnesses
4. Factors influencing the dynamics of insulin action, such as exercise, injection site, temperature of the environment, etc.
5. Emotional factors

requires calm management. Anxiety usually leads to an increase in the brittleness.

Marital Stress

Management of diabetes can cause stress in a marriage. A wife who does not have diabetes has the challenge of helping her husband follow his meal plan. This means planning and preparing meals carefully. It will mean adjusting the serving time to his blood glucose level, which may not be known until a few minutes before the normal mealtime. If his blood glucose is high, he may say, "I'd better wait to eat for about an hour until I get my blood glucose under better control." Wives often find such demands frustrating, especially when he doesn't try to help her plan more efficiently.

When the wife has diabetes, the husband may find the carefully planned meals irritating. He may want to be supportive, but resent frequent changes in meal schedules.

When early signs of hypoglycemia appear, the spouse will frequently tell his or her diabetic partner, "Honey, I think you need to eat." Such logical advice is sometimes rejected angrily, "I am all right. Leave me alone!" A bitter argument may follow. Almost always, the spouse proves to be correct. After the diabetic spouse eats some food, the couple calms down, even though the pain from the emotional encounter may last for hours or even days. People often do not realize what they are saying during hypoglycemia. The emotional outburst often includes sarcastic and hateful remarks, which are really not rational. The brain doesn't function normally on too little glucose. The consequences of a hypoglycemic confrontation are often painful and may be difficult to forget quickly. Often the diabetic seems to think, "Why all the fuss! It's over now. I'm sorry." The spouse may not be so forgiving when the episodes seem to occur with unnecessary frequency.

Various studies have shown that diabetes can affect the emotional well-being of the other family members. The effect of hypoglycemia can be temporarily negative, but such episodes are just as likely to increase family cohesion and solidarity. Family members realize that arguments over details of the diabetes management effort are seldom productive. Calm discussion most often yields peaceful planning, and everyone gains.

Depression

Depression is a serious illness that may be precipitated by discouragement over the many life adjustments that all people with diabetes must make. Of course, we are also vulnerable to all the normal stresses that precipitate depression. Depression is much more common in people who have serious physical illness. It has been reported to be detected in about 10% of general outpatients in clinics and in 22–33% of inpatients in hospitals. The normal frequency of depression in the general population is about 4%. In people with diabetes, depression has been reported to be as high as 18% and is more common in women. Individuals who have widely fluctuating blood glucose levels and frequent hypoglycemic attacks certainly experience increased stress and may fall into a depression.

Guilt feelings can cause depression or, at least, pessimistic moods. When complications appear, people with diabetes often feel that if they had been more careful, they would not have the difficulty they have now. Relatives can also get discouraged. Dr. Lincoln's father told him during the months after the diagnosis was first made, "I'll make it up to you somehow." The implication was that it was his fault that diabetes had developed in his son. There was no family history of diabetes, but somehow he felt that he had done something wrong. Since there is a strong genetic component in this disease, diabetic parents often feel guilty when they have a child who develops diabetes, too.

None of us want to "give" diabetes to our children or grandchildren. We do want to give life and love and a chance to pursue the joys and troubles that are part of our human condition. If you have diabetes and your child or grandchild develops diabetes, forget guilt and choose to offer your love, support, and experience as a gift that will make adjustment to living with diabetes easier for him or her. Rejoice in the gift of life even if you have diabetes. Share with the child that learning to control diabetes will also serve him or her well in solving life's other problems.

The support role

Although physicians are busy and usually have little time to chat with their patients, they should show interest in the patient's personal problems and concerns about diabetes. This can be a great help. When a young person with diabetes has achieved slightly better control and seems to be developing confidence and more independence, compliments from the family and health team members can be very beneficial. Family members should realize that depression is more common in people with diabetes of all ages and encourage their loved ones to seek counseling when they seem to be depressed.

There appears to be little information on suicides in diabetics. You may wonder if anyone ever uses excess insulin to commit suicide. It would be an extremely inefficient method. Insulin takes a long time to kill, and the victim would usually have been found and taken to a hospital where treatment, even for those who have been unconscious for many hours, is remarkably effective.

Memory loss and depression

When older people with diabetes experience longer lasting and more severe confusion and short-term memory loss following episodes of hypoglycemia, they may panic. They may suffer from depression, thinking that permanent brain damage has occurred. The depression that accompanies memory loss makes the memory loss worse. Once the depression is relieved and time passes, most people find that their memory improves to about the same level as could be expected in any person of the same age. Most people, whether or not they have diabetes, have some memory loss with aging. Even if the hundreds of episodes of hypoglycemia during a lifetime of tight control of diabetes eventually cause a mild loss of short-term memory, it is a small price to pay for survival and avoidance of other debilitating complications of diabetes.

Depression can destroy the delicate balance you have achieved while performing your daily diabetic routine. It can creep up on you. If you develop several of the signs and symptoms of depression in Table 18-2 and they persist for more than a week or two, you should consider seeking the help of your physician.

When depressed, most of us who live with diabetes lose the motivation and discipline to keep our blood sugar in good control. When we lose control of blood sugar, we feel physically and mentally ill. This contributes to a deeper sense of depression. Be alert for the warning signs of depression. Medication and counseling can relieve the symptoms, so you can resume your diabetes management and return to good health.

TABLE 18-2

Signs of Depression

1. Loss of interest in pleasurable activities

2. Sleep disturbance

3. Increase or decrease of usual appetite

4. Loss of usual energy

5. Depressed mood

6. Crying spells

7. Thoughts of suicide

8. Feelings of worthlessness

19

Losing Awareness of Hypoglycemia

Not recognizing your early symptoms of low blood sugar is a serious problem. It is sometimes called "hypoglycemia unawareness." It is more accurate to call it reduced hypoglycemia awareness. After 10–20 years on insulin treatment, most people with diabetes will have an occasional problem of reduced awareness, and a few may become almost totally unaware of the early symptoms of hypoglycemia.

When your brain doesn't get enough glucose, as always happens during hypoglycemia, there are a wide variety of symptoms that can develop. These include an inner trembling, sweating, fatigue, irritability, bizarre behavior, weakness, dizziness, clumsiness, and many others. Confusion and difficulty in speaking, reading, and thinking appear. There is no characteristic pattern. This great variety of symptoms occurs because hypoglycemia affects the thinking centers of the brain. As a consequence, these symptoms collectively are called neuroglycopenia, which means symptoms caused by the brain not having enough glucose.

The problem is that one time you might get a headache, another time double vision, another time hunger, and another time you might just get quiet and confused. Probably the most consistent symptom is an inner tremulousness or anxiety.

Unfortunately, after you have had many hypoglycemic episodes and have had diabetes for 10–20 years, early symptoms of low blood glucose are harder to recognize. When they first appear, they are so mild that they are often easy to ignore, especially if you are busy. Also, as the blood glucose continues to fall, the brain functions more and more poorly, so you can't recognize the symptoms. You become so increasingly dull and slow that you may not realize that you are behaving strangely. In most cases when the symptoms get more severe, the person recognizes the problem and gets something to eat. In some cases, the person still does not recognize the problem, and another person may have to get you to eat something.

The wife of a retired insurance salesman who had had diabetes for more than 30 years reported, "I can tell when my husband needs to eat when he comes home from work. He looks funny. He is pale, and his eyes are beady. If he labors over the mail and just shuffles through it and seems to get nowhere, I will get him some orange juice, and usually he will drink it. He does not seem to have any idea that his blood sugar is low. Sometimes he gets argumentative."

Sometimes your reduced awareness may actually be a subconscious suppression of symptoms in order to complete a task. If you are busy and don't want to be interrupted, it is easy to ignore the early symptoms and consciously or unconsciously tell yourself, "I'll finish what I am doing, and then I'll go get something to eat." If you are mowing the lawn and seem to be getting tired earlier than usual, you may push on and try to finish the job, not realizing that your problem is hypoglycemia and not fatigue.

If your glucose level is dropping to a very low level and you need to perform thinking or problem-solving functions, you are much more likely to realize that something is wrong. When the brain is "coasting" and not being challenged, then hypoglycemia is likely to sneak up on you.

Being asleep is a common form of unawareness. People who sleep lightly may be awakened by the slightest change in the environment in the room or by a mild disturbance in bodily function. More commonly, people sleep very soundly and are not awakened by considerable commotion in their bedroom or by mild internal disturbances such as a headache. Most severe episodes of hypoglycemia that require someone else to administer food to you occur at night while you are sleeping. Most physicians do not include hypoglycemic episodes that occur during sleep as examples of unawareness. An episode that is due to lack of awareness is one that occurs while you are awake.

We don't know how widespread lack of awareness of the symptoms of hypoglycemia is. Experts speculate that 1/3 to 1/2 of all people who use insulin have some difficulty with lack of awareness. In one study, 9 out of 10 people who did not have diabetes recognized symptoms of hypoglycemia when their blood glucose was artificially lowered to 45 mg/dl, but only 4 out of 15 people with diabetes recognized their symptoms.

If you have severe difficulty in recognizing early symptoms of hypoglycemia, your target blood glucose levels may have to be raised and your blood glucose allowed to stay in a higher range.

Increasing your awareness

Is there any way to increase your awareness? It would seem logical to suggest that if you always wrote down what you thought your blood glucose was going to be before you checked it, you might be able to sharpen your awareness. There has been some success in such attempts, but they have generally been disappointing. It is extremely difficult to predict what your blood glucose will be just by how you feel, even if you only attempt to predict whether you are high (over 150 mg/dl), medium (75–150 mg/dl), or low (less than 75 mg/dl). Most people will be disappointed at how poorly they guess. When your glucose is extremely high (over 300 mg/dl) or extremely low (50 mg/dl), your prediction is usually much better. The accuracy of your prediction improves if your estimate is also based on recalling the time of your previous insulin dose (quantity and time), the last food you ate (quality and quantity), and your most recent exercise (intensity and duration).

If you try to keep your blood glucose low (less than 100 mg/dl) all the time, you tend to reduce awareness. The brain needs to "see" various levels in order to keep a perspective as to what is too low. Allowing an occasional high, for example from 150–200 mg/dl, for a couple of hours is not harmful and still allows for a low HbA1c level (chapter 4).

If your life depended on not becoming hypoglycemic during the next 8 hours and you were not allowed to eat enough to keep your blood glucose continuously high, you could probably do reasonably well by constantly being alert to the earliest symptoms of hypoglycemia. The difficulty is that this level of surveillance is just not possible as a way of life. You are like everybody else. You are busy and preoccupied with hundreds of things. You don't have the time, energy, or inclination to look constantly for hypoglycemia signals. Hypoglycemia unawareness typically occurs on an average day when everything seems to be perfectly normal. The low blood glucose "just crept up on me. I guess I wasn't paying attention."

There doesn't appear to be any easy way to increase your awareness. That doesn't mean that there aren't some tricks that you can use during times when awareness is particularly important. The most obvious time is when you are driving and when you are alone. A spouse or family member usually is keenly sensitive to changes in your behavior that suggest that you might be hypoglycemic. A list of possible ways to increase awareness is given in Table 19-1. You may have developed your own tricks, and this table gives you a few of ours.

If you have many episodes of hypoglycemia, this may reduce the release of counter-regulatory hormones, such as epinephrine and glucagon (chapter 1), that are the main defenses against hypoglycemia. Patients who have been under poor control tend to have hypoglycemic symptoms at a higher blood glucose level than those under tight control. Healthy people who don't have diabetes have been studied to see what happens to them when they are subjected to a series of hypoglycemic episodes. After four episodes, a lower level of glucose was required to cause symptoms of hypoglycemia. Apparently the brain gets accustomed to hypoglycemia and tolerates it better, delaying the appearance of symptoms.

TABLE 19-1

Ways to Increase Awareness of Hypoglycemia

1. Monitor blood glucose frequently, especially before driving and during long trips.

2. When driving long distances alone, periodically try some mental exercise that puts considerable demand on memory or intelligence. For example, add up the numbers on your odometer twice, from left to right and right to left, to see if you get the same answer.

3. Monitor your thinking capacity, especially during times when you expect your blood glucose to be on the low side.

4. If you start making mistakes in routine physical or mental activities, remind yourself that this may be a sign of hypoglycemia and do something about it right then.

5. Watch out for times when you seem to be quiet and withdrawn or silly and unusually talkative.

6. Irritability and impatience may be early signs of hypoglycemia.

7. When you seem to be getting unusually tired, you may be becoming hypoglycemic.

8. Challenge yourself to rapidly read a paragraph or two in a newspaper and see if you can understand it. If not, suspect hypoglycemia.

9. Avoid keeping your blood glucose within too narrow a range. Allow occasional highs in the 200 mg/dl range for a few hours. The brain needs to "see" various levels in order to keep a perspective as to what is high and what is low.

20

Managing Your
Own Diabetes

Since you will have to treat your disease for the rest of your life, you need to develop a personal philosophy about how you are going to manage your treatment. The first impulse of people who are newly diagnosed is to depend on their physicians to tell them exactly what to do. This is because with most diseases, physicians prescribe medications, diets, changes in lifestyle, physical therapy, and occasionally recommend surgery. Patients expect to follow their physician's instructions.

A general plan for diet, insulin or oral medications, and exercise can be prescribed by a physician, but it will not result in good blood glucose control unless it is skillfully implemented by you. Even if you are an extremely disciplined person and follow diet instructions, insulin dosage, and exercise advice to the letter, your blood glucose levels are likely to vary widely. You have to live your life pretty much like everyone else. Going to school, working, playing, having a family, and experiencing stress are little different for you than for your relatives and friends. The treatment of diabetes has to follow the particulars of each person's career, family life, and lifestyle.

It is extremely difficult to follow a rigid meal plan. With tight schedules and demands to get jobs done on time, it is even harder to eat meals at the same time each day. Because many people travel long distances to school or work, delays due to traffic jams or weather often prevent following an eating schedule. New guidelines in the dietary management of diabetes allow much more flexibility in preparing meals or eating in fast-food restaurants. Especially with the use of the new rapid-acting insulin before each meal, it is possible to make sudden adjustments in how much and when you eat.

Physical fitness and athletic achievements are an important part of diabetes management for young, middle-aged, and older people. Exercise burns calories, so you require less insulin. Prescribing precise amounts of exercise is nearly impossible because the expenditure of calories varies with each person and with the vigor and duration of the exercise. No physician can possibly prescribe how vigorously young people should play their chosen sports or how fast middle-aged and older people should jog or walk.

Because of these and other uncertainties, you have no choice but to learn how to manage your own diabetes. To learn how to do this requires some expert help. Unfortunately, in a nationwide study of people with diabetes, 41% with type 1 diabetes, 51% with insulin-treated type 2, and 76% with type 2 who did not take insulin reported that they had never received any training. They never attended a diabetes education class or any other education program. If you have never received any training, even though you think you are doing reasonably well now, you need to go back and learn the basics. If your physician can't refer you to a local training program, you can contact the regional office of the American Diabetes Association closest to you or the National Office at 1701 N. Beauregard Street, Alexandria, VA 22311 or call 1-800-DIABETES (342-2383).

The ADA Web site is www.diabetes.org. If there are few or no education programs in your area, the ADA has many books to help you educate yourself further. *Diabetes Forecast* magazine is very helpful at keeping you advised of the latest developments and helping you refine your technique of basic management.

By measuring your own blood glucose levels at least four times a day, you will gradually learn how your food intake, insulin dose, and exercise affect your blood glucose. You will gradually learn how to manage your disease. It is a slow process, and you will make mistakes. Like learning a new sport or dance, coaching plus practice are the secrets for success. Physicians and diabetes educators can be your coaches. Parents, spouses, relatives, friends, and other people with diabetes can be your cheerleaders and supporters. But you have to run the race, play the game, dance the dance yourself! In other words, you and only you can manage your own disease. Good luck! We know that you can do it.

Index

SMBG. *See* Self-monitoring blood glucose
Sodas
sweetened, to treat hypoglycemia, 35, 42
Sprains and strains, 13
Stress. *See also* Depression in diabetes
help from exercise, 68
marital, 137–138
memory loss and, 140–141
signs of, 141
support role in, 139–140
Sucrose tablets, gels, or liquids to treat hypoglycemia, 42
Sugar. *See* Blood glucose
Sugar cubes
to treat hypoglycemia, 36
Support role
with depression in diabetes, 139–140
Symptoms of hypoglycemia, 3–4, 71–72, 128–141

T

Teenagers. *See* Adolescents
Time consumed by blood glucose monitoring, 20
Timing food
for the blood sugar blues in school, 77
Traveling and hypoglycemia, 92, 108–113
checklist for, 111

Treating hypoglycemia, 6–7, 32–43, 40–43
amount to eat, 38–39
cautions with alcohol use, 43
follow up to glucagon administration, 42–43
foods to use, 34–37
at home, 33–39
individual factors, 37–38
severe, 40–43
using glucagon, 41–42
Types of insulin
effects on insulin action, 49–50

U

UKPDS. *See* United Kingdom Prospective Diabetes Study (UKPDS)
Unconsciousness, 43, 91, 128
United Kingdom Prospective Diabetes Study (UKPDS), 11–12

V

Vision
effects of hypoglycemia on, 128–132

W

Warmth
effects on insulin action, 46–47

About the American Diabetes Association

The American Diabetes Association is the nation's leading voluntary health organization supporting diabetes research, information, and advocacy. Its mission is to prevent and cure diabetes and to improve the lives of all people affected by diabetes. The American Diabetes Association is the leading publisher of comprehensive diabetes information. Its huge library of practical and authoritative books for people with diabetes covers every aspect of self-care—cooking and nutrition, fitness, weight control, medications, complications, emotional issues, and general self-care.

To order American Diabetes Association books: Call 1-800-232-6733. http://store.diabetes.org [Note: there is no need to use www when typing this particular Web address]

To join the American Diabetes Association: Call 1-800-806-7801. www.diabetes.org/membership

For more information about diabetes or ADA programs and services: Call 1-800-342-2383. E-mail: Customerservice@diabetes.org www.diabetes.org

To locate an ADA/NCQA Recognized Provider of quality diabetes care in your area: Call 1-703-549-1500 ext. 2202. www.diabetes.org/recognition/Physicians/ListAll.asp

To find an ADA Recognized Education Program in your area: Call 1-888-232-0822. www.diabetes.org/recognition/education.asp

To join the fight to increase funding for diabetes research, end discrimination, and improve insurance coverage: Call 1-800-342-2383. www.diabetes.org/advocacy

To find out how you can get involved with the programs in your community: Call 1-800-342-2383. See below for program Web addresses.

- American Diabetes Month: Educational activities aimed at those diagnosed with diabetes—month of November. www.diabetes.org/ADM
- American Diabetes Alert: Annual public awareness campaign to find the undiagnosed—held the fourth Tuesday in March. www.diabetes.org/alert
- The Diabetes Assistance & Resources Program (DAR): diabetes awareness program targeted to the Latino community. www.diabetes.org/DAR
- African American Program: diabetes awareness program targeted to the African American community. www.diabetes.org/africanamerican
- Awakening the Spirit: Pathways to Diabetes Prevention & Control: diabetes awareness program targeted to the Native American community. www.diabetes.org/awakening

To find out about an important research project regarding type 2 diabetes: www.diabetes.org/ada/research.asp

To obtain information on making a planned gift or charitable bequest: Call 1-888-700-7029. www.diabetes.org/ada/plan.asp

To make a donation or memorial contribution: Call 1-800-342-2383. www.diabetes.org/ada/cont.asp